Clinical
IVF Forum

Current Views in
Assisted Reproduction

Edited by
Phillip L. Matson
and
Brian A. Lieberman

Manchester University Press
Manchester and New York
Distributed exclusively in the USA and Canada by St. Martin's Press

Published by Manchester University Press
Oxford Road, Manchester M13 9PL, UK
and Room 400, 175 Fifth Avenue,
New York, NY 10010, USA

Distributed exclusively in the USA and Canada
by St. Martin's Press, Inc.,
175 Fifth Avenue, New York, NY 10010, USA

British Library cataloguing in publication data
Clinical IVF forum.
    1. Man. In vitro conception
    I. Matson, Phillip L. II. Lieberman, Brian A.
    618.178059

Library of Congress Cataloging in Publication Data applied for

ISBN 0-7190-3410-8 paperback

Typeset in Great Britain by
Breeze Ltd, Manchester

Printed in Great Britain
by Biddles Ltd, Guildford and King's Lynn

Proceedings of a
Serono Seminar
held during
9th & 10th March 1990
Presented with the Compliments of
Serono Laboratories (UK) Ltd
99 Bridge Road East, Welwyn Garden City, Hertfordshire AL7 1BG

Contents

Page

Preface   v
Contributors   vii

Chapter No.

1 *R. Fleming, M.E. Jamieson, J.R.T. Coutts*   1
   The Use of GnRH-Analogs in Assisted Reproduction

2 *Z.H.Z. Ibrahim, P. Buck, P.L. Matson, B.A. Lieberman*   20
   Inclusion of Human Growth Hormone (hGH) in Stimulation
   Regimens for Poor Responders

3 *S. Fishel, S. Antinori, J. Webster*   29
   Evaluation of the Inclusion of FSH in Follicular Stimulation
   Regimes

4 *C. Howles*   41
   GnRH Analogues, Past Present and Future Uses in Superovulation Regimens

5 *D.H. Barlow, D. Egan, C. Ross*   63
   The Outcome of IVF Pregnancy

6 *S.W. D'Souza, E. Rivlin, P. Buck, B.A. Lieberman*   70
   Children Conceived by in Vitro Fertilization

7 *I. Craft*   79
   A Flexible Approach to Assisted Conception

8 *Revd. Dr. T. Appleton*   93
   Dealing with Failure in an Assisted Reproduction Programme

9   *B.E. Talansky, H.E. Malter, A. Adler, M. Alikani, A. Berkeley,*   101
    O. Davis, M. Graf, A. Reing, Z. Rosenwaks, J. Cohen
    Limitations of Zona Pellucida Micromanipulation in the
    Human

10 *P.L. Matson*   112
    The Usefulness of IVF, GIFT and IUI in the Treatment of Male
    Infertility

11 *W.C.L. Ford*   123
    The Role of Oxygen Free Radicals in the Pathology of
    Human Spermatozoa: Implications for IVF

12 *A. Isidori*   140
    Gonadotrophin Therapy in the Male

Preface

The painstaking and pioneering research undertaken by the late Patrick Steptoe and Professor Robert Edwards in Oldham, Lancashire, was rewarded by the birth of Louise Brown and as a direct consequence of their efforts, in vitro fertilization is now accepted as an established medical practice. The technique has, throughout the world, helped thousands of infertile couples and the associated and continuing research and development has added significantly to our knowledge and understanding of human reproduction and reproductive disorders.

It was thought appropriate to invite experts in the field of assisted reproduction to the North West of England where it all began, to present their current views on topics of interest. This book is a record of their contributions at the meeting held at the Hilton Hotel, Manchester in March 1990 and we hope that it will prove of value to workers in this field.

Pituitary down-regulation with GnRH agonists prior to ovarian stimulation with human menopausal gonadotrophin is associated with a high rate of implantation and fewer women are now discharged from treatment because of an inappropriate LH surge. However this is accompanied by high rates of multiple implantations and ovarian hyperstimulation. The current state of GnRH agonists is discussed in detail by Dr Richard Fleming. Approximately 10% of women respond inadequately to induction of ovulation and the endeavours of the Manchester group to augment the ovarian response to hMG by human growth hormone is discussed by Dr Zaky Ibrahim. The outcome of treatment using different regimes is compared by Dr Simon Fishel and the role of GnRH agonists and antagonists is further discussed by Dr Colin Howles.

The outcome of pregnancies achieved by assisted reproduction is discussed in two complimentary chapters by Drs David Barlow and Stephen D'Souza. This audit is fundamental to the continuation of IVF programmes and provides essential data for the counselling of prospective couples.

The arguments in favour of a flexible approach in assisted reproduction are presented by Professor Ian Craft. Unfortunately assisted reproduction still fails more often than it succeeds and Rev. Dr Tim Appleton discusses counselling after failed treatment.

Whilst in general there are rational and, in many instances, highly successful therapies available for the treatment of female infertility, the same cannot be said for sperm disorders. Dr Jacques Cohen discusses the latest data using oocyte micromanipulation and partial zona dissection. The role of assisted reproduction in the treatment of male disorders is analysed by Dr Phillip Matson. The role of oxygen free radicals as a basis for male disorders is advanced by Dr Christopher Ford, and Professor Aldo Isidori concludes by discussing the role of gonadotrophin therapy in the male.

Brian Lieberman
Phillip Matson

Contributors

A. Adler. The Centre for Reproductive Medicine and Infertility, Department of Obstetrics and Gynaecology, Cornell University Medical College, New York, USA.

M. Alikani. The Centre for Reproductive Medicine and Infertility, Department of Obstetrics and Gynaecology, Cornell University Medical College, New York, USA.

S. Antinori. Rapru, Clinica Nomentana, Via Guattani - 4, Rome, Italy.

T. Appleton. Infertility Support Counselling, 44 Eversden Road, Harlton Cambridge CB3 7ET, UK.

D. Barlow. Nuffield Department of Obstetrics and Gynaecology, John Radcliffe Hospital, Oxford, UK.

A. Berkeley. The Centre for Reproductive Medicine and Infertility, Department of Obstetrics and Gynaecology, Cornell University Medical College, New York, USA.

P. Buck. Regional IVF Unit, St. Mary's Hospital, Manchester M13 0JH, UK.

J. Cohen. The Centre for Reproductive Medicine and Infertility, Department of Obstetrics and Gynaecology, Cornell University Medical College, New York, USA.

J.R.T. Coutts. University Department of Obstetrics and Gynaecology, Royal Infirmary, Glasgow, G31 2ER, UK.

I. Craft. London Fertility Centre, Cozens House, 112A Harley Street, London W1N 1AF, UK.

O. Davis. The Centre for Reproductive Medicine and Infertility, Department of Obstetrics and Gynaecology, Cornell University Medical College, New York, USA.

S. W. D'Souza. Department of Child Health, St Mary's Hospital, Manchester M13 0JH, UK.

D. Egan. Nuffield Department of Obstetrics and Gynaecology, John Radcliffe Hospital, Oxford, UK.

S. Fishel. Department of Obstetrics and Gynaecology, University of Nottingham; and The Park Hospital, Sherwood Lodge Drive,Arnold, Nottingham NG5 8RX, UK.

R. Fleming. University Department of Obstetrics and Gynaecology, Royal Infirmary, Glasgow G31 2ER, UK.

W.C.L. Ford. University Department of Obstetrics and Gynaecology, Bristol Maternity Hospital, Bristol BS2 8EG, UK.

M. Graf. The Centre for Reproductive Medicine and Infertility, Department of Obstetrics and Gynaecology, Cornell University Medical College, New York, USA.

C. Howles. Serono Labs (UK) Ltd., Welwyn Garden City, UK.

Z.H.Z. Ibrahim. Regional IVF Unit, St Mary's Hospital, Manchester M13 0JH, UK.

A. Isidori. Chair of Andrology, University of Rome, Rome, Italy.

M.E. Jamieson. University Department of Obstetrics and Gynaecology, Royal Infirmary, Glasgow, G31 2ER, UK.

B.A. Lieberman. Regional IVF Unit, St Mary's Hospital, Manchester M13 0JH, UK.

H.E. Malter. The Centre for Reproductive Medicine and Infertility, Department of Obstetrics and Gynaecology, Cornell University Medical College, New York, USA.

P.L. Matson. Regional IVF Unit, St Mary's Hospital, Manchester M13 0JH, UK.

A. Reing. The Centre for Reproductive Medicine and Infertility, Department of Obstetrics and Gynaecology, Cornell University Medical College, New York, USA.

E. Rivlin. Department of Child Psychology, St Mary's Hospital, Manchester M13 0JH. UK.

C. Ross. Nuffield Department of Obstetrics and Gynaecology, John Radcliffe Hospital, Oxford, UK.

Z. Rosenwaks. The Centre for Reproductive Medicine and Infertility, Department of Obstetrics and Gynaecology, Cornell University Medical College, New York, USA.

B.E. Talansky. The Centre for Reproductive Medicine and Infertility, Department of Obstetrics and Gynaecology, Cornell University Medical College, New York, USA.

J. Webster. The Park Hospital, Sherwood Lodge Drive, Arnold, Nottingham NG5 8RX, UK.

1 *R. Fleming, M.E.Jamieson, J.R.T. Coutts*

THE USE OF GnRH-ANALOGS IN ASSISTED REPRODUCTION

Introduction

There is abundant evidence from IVF and GIFT centres around the world indicating the benefits of multiple gametes available for processing. The more oocytes available, the more embryos there will be for transfer, and the higher the pregnancy rate. The more embryos available for cryopreservation, the better the chances of subsequent survival and replacement. Therefore, multiple follicular development is essential for a successful assisted conception programme.

The vast majority of patients in IVF/GIFT programmes have normal menstrual rhythm with implicit normal ovarian and pituitary function; both of which are designed to produce a single dominant follicle and oocyte each month. Obtaining multiple follicular growth requires pharmacological manipulation of ovarian metabolism, and complicating factors may arise from both ovarian and pituitary sources. The number and variety of methods used to achieve multiple follicular growth are testament to the needs to find a simple, cheap and effective regimen with negligible complication rates.

The GnRH-Analogs (GnRH-A) are able to both stimulate and suppress gonadotrophin output, and both of these qualities may be exploited in attempts to achieve controlled ovarian stimulation without undesirable pituitary intervention. The short term response to treatment with a GnRH-A is acute release of LH and FSH to concentrations seen during the mid-cycle LH surge, while continued frequent administration results in suppression of LH to concentrations close to the limits of specific radioimmunoassay sensitivity. Figure 1 shows the effect of protracted treatment with buserelin (by intra nasal spray; Hoechst UK Ltd.) in women with normal and with elevated LH at the start of treatment. Following the 'flare' effect, the concentration of LH returned to pre-treatment levels in 4-6 days,

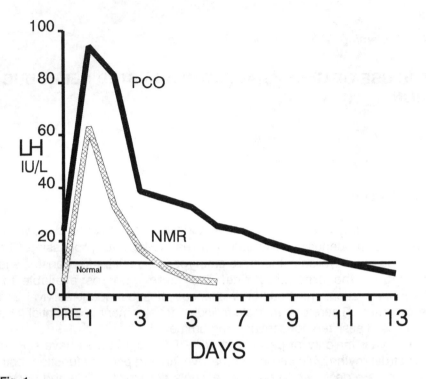

Fig. 1.
LH responses to continued treatment with a GnRH-A in women with normal menstrual rhythm (NMR) and with oligomenorrhoea and elevated LH (PCO).

and continued to decline thereafter. The patients with PCO syndrome (elevated LH at the start) required a further 10 days treatment to suppress the LH to low-normal levels. The net result of this action is the suppression of ovarian function for the duration of treatment, and this phenomenon has lead to the abundant clinical applications of GnRH-As in gynaecology. However, it is the ability to suppress LH activity during the period of follicular maturation that has lead to the application in IVF/GIFT programmes.

Aspects of Follicular Growth

In the normal cycling woman there is a steady turnover of follicles from primordial through primary to Graafian follicle and to atresia (Gougeon and Lefebre, 1983). Each month one exceptional follicle escapes this fate by responding to the premenstrual rise in FSH with increased estradiol (E2) biosynthesis and growth, and while it proceeds to maturity the other follicles at apparently similar stages of development continue to undergo atresia: probably because of reduced pituitary output of FSH following the negative feedback effect of the increased concentrations of plasma E2. Actively increasing follicular stimulation either with anti-estrogens and/or exogenous gonadotrophins (HMG) in the early and mid follicular phase prevents or rescues a number of the follicles from atresia and stimulates a cohort through the latter stages of maturation. In this way a number of follicles can be brought to apparent maturity simultaneously. However, the continued elevations of FSH through the follicular phase continues to recruit follicles from subsequent cohorts and this produces a broad spectrum of follicle size (maturity). This is a potential problem which may have no simple solution.

Immature follicles are exclusively FSH sensitive, but as they grow their ability to respond to LH increases even at relatively small and early stages of development. Thus the timing of the luteinizing signal is important; and the ovary should only be exposed to it when a discreet number of follicles is mature.

The best estimate of individual follicle maturity is its diameter (FD), and in the normal cycle the FD on the day of the LH surge lies between 17 and 25 mm with a mean of 20 mm (Hackeloer et al, 1979). Accordingly, the luteinizing signal (HCG) should be administered (Day 0) when at least one FD is at 20 mm with a small number in the "mature" size range. Interestingly, this does not mean that follicles with smaller FDs will not yield oocytes capable of establishing a pregnancy, although in general, the chances of obtaining good embryo development are better with oocytes from larger follicles (Jamieson et al, 1988). Of course, all this assumes that no LH surge has taken place to luteinize the follicles prior to HCG administration, and no other complicating factors have intervened.

The Role of LH

When studying LH data in the follicular phase of stimulated cycles there may be a problem in distinguishing between basally elevated concentrations and those deriving from attenuated LH surges. Figure 2 shows the responses to HMG of a patient with normal menstrual rhythm, who showed an LH surge well before any follicle attained the mature size range. It elicited a substantial rise in plasma progesterone (P) concentrations

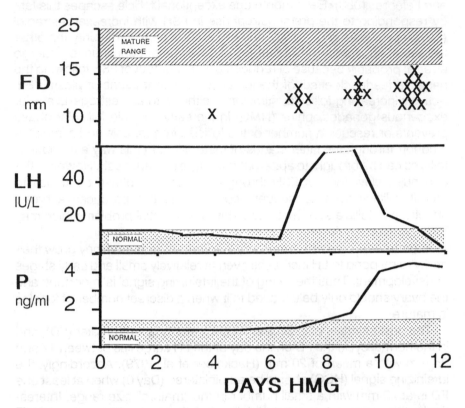

Fig. 2.
An example of pre-HCG (premature) luteinization in a patient treated with HMG alone. The LH surge and the rise in P occurred well before any follicle (X) achieved the 'mature size' range.

before HCG could be administered in accordance with the established criteria for Day 0 (>2 mature sized follicles). The LH concentrations prior to the surge were well within the normal range.

It is possible that high basal LH concentrations, as those found in patients with PCO, may have direct negative influences upon oocyte viability (Stanger and Yovich, 1985; Howles et al, 1986), although other evidence has failed to determine any direct evidence in support of this (Thomas et al, 1989). On the other hand, LH surges as in Figure 2, undoubtedly have direct effects which induce luteinization and initiate the processes of ovulation in follicles mature enough to respond. When an LH surge is detected, and the cohort of follicles is mature enough the IVF/GIFT procedure may continue with or without HCG as "back-up"

(Edwards and Steptoe, 1975). However, the undetected LH surge and/or the surge at inappropriate levels of follicular development are events with direct detrimental effects (Fleming and Coutts, 1986), even if pre-operative ovulation does not take place (Stanger and Yovich, 1984).

In ovulation induction, the premature LH surge renders the whole treatment cycle redundant, and in cases when the LH surge occurs at the time HCG would have been withheld due to over-response, it can prove disastrous because of multiple ovulation. The spontaneous LH surge has been reported to occur in more than 30% of cycles treated with HMG alone prior to the identification of a single mature-sized follicle (Fleming and Coutts, 1986). In cycles treated with Clomid and HMG in an IVF pro-gramme, more than 40% of cycles showed LH surges prior to HCG (Hillier et al, 1985). These data alone argue the case for development of protocols which suppress endogenous LH throughout the late follicular phase; particularly in centres not equipped with rapid access to operating fa-cilities.

It may be that the "high basal" levels of LH detected in the studies reported above (Stanger and Yovich, 1985; Howles et al, 1986) represent grouped data showing attenuated LH surges (Messinis et al, 1986), and so both approaches are, in fact, observing the same physiological event: increased LH activity and influence upon follicles at inappropriate stages of development. Whatever the explanation, monitoring of responses would be simplified without interference from LH during follicular stimula-tion, and for this reason GnRH-Analogs have been taken up enthusiasti-cally and effectively in many centres.

Pre-HCG Luteinization

The primary marker of an effective LH surge at any stage is luteinization and a rise in peripheral P concentrations. This can be used to detect the pre-HCG LH surge, but its effects at the level of the endometrium may be just as important as its effects on the follicle. There is no doubt that the oestrogenised endometrium can respond to moderate elevations in P by transforming from proliferative to secretory, but the minimum concentra-tions required to effect this change are unknown. The effects of advancing the stage of endometrial development ahead of embryo development would lead to an asynchrony which may cause failure of viable implanta-tion.

One consequence of an LH surge ocurring before the criteria for HCG administration are established is ovulation prior to oocyte retrieval. When

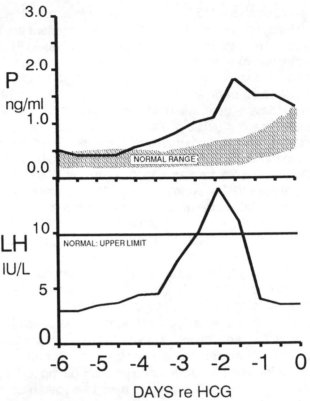

Fig. 3.
Mean profiles of P and LH from cycles (n = 14) with post-mature oocytes. The P profile is superimposed on the laboratory normal cycle ranges and shows elevations starting at day -4. The LH profile is compared with the normal cycle follicular phase upper limit.

this happens, there is a tendency for only the more mature follicles (FD > 16mm) to release their oocytes, while the smaller follicles tend to entrap them (Stanger and Yovich, 1984), although retrieval by aspiration may be effective. This results in a reduced supply of oocytes whose ability to fertilize and yield viable embryos may be compromised.

A secondary observation in cycles treated with HMG alone is that of oocyte post-maturity (PM), which are identified by their granular appearance in combination with a disintegrated, friable collection of cumulus cells. These PM oocytes are usually found associated with apparently normal oocytes, but in cycles with reduced fertilization rates and low pregnancy potential. Retrospective hormone analyses of cycles with PM oocytes is shown in Fig. 3. and they demonstrate mean data which

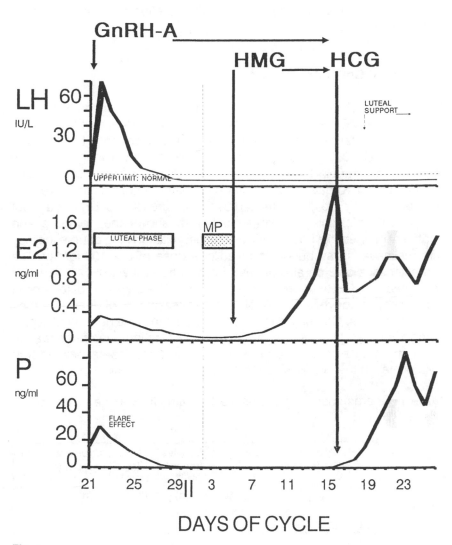

Fig. 4.
LH, E2 and P profiles of a typical patient's response to the long course GnRH-A/HMG treatment protocol with initiation of GNRH-A in the mid-luteal phase of the cycle prior to HMG treatment.

disguise the fact that each cycle showed an LH surge (attenuated) more than 24h before the LH surge, and moderate elevations in P which were close to the 1.5 ng/ml concentration in 2 successive samples which would have elicited cycle cancellation. Again, it is not clear whether the low pregnancy potential of these cycles is due to effects at the follicular or endometrial level.

Influence of GnRH-As

The original publication of the use of GnRH-As during induction of follicular growth with HMG was in women with normal menstrual rhythm and the GnRH-A was started in the luteal phase of the cycle prior to treatment (Fleming et al, 1982). This has now become known as a 'long course' as in cycles with the GnRH-A started on cycle day 1 and the HMG therapy started at least 10 days later or after demonstration of full "down-regulation" of LH. They are characterized by the suppression of LH throughout the phase of follicular growth, and Fig. 4. shows the hormone and treatment profiles of a patient on luteal phase initiated long course therapy with the nasal spray buserelin given at a dose of 5 x 100ug/day. The characteristics of 2 parallel series of cycles treated with HMG alone or combined with GnRH-A are shown in Table 1. There was no difference in the number of oocytes (or their subjective assessment of quality) or their fertilization rates. The major differences were seen in the number of cycles failing to proceed to OR due to pre-HCG luteinization, the concentration of LH at the time of HCG, and the elimination of cycles associated with PM oocytes in the GnRH-A group.

Table 1. Characteristics of cycles treated with HMG alone or combined with GnRH-A.

Treatment	Cycle Starts	OR		Oocytes (mean/ OR)	LH (at HCG)	Cycles with PM oocytes	
	(n)	(n)	(%)	(n)	(IU/L)	(n)	(%)
HMG	75	51	68	7.4	4.8	10	19.6
GnRH-A + HMG	32	32	100	7.0	1.4 *	0	0

* P < 0.001

Fig. 5. shows the hormone profiles leading to HCG administration of 2 similar series of IVF patients and demonstrates that although there was no difference in the P profiles (cycles with P > 1.5 mg/ml were disconti-

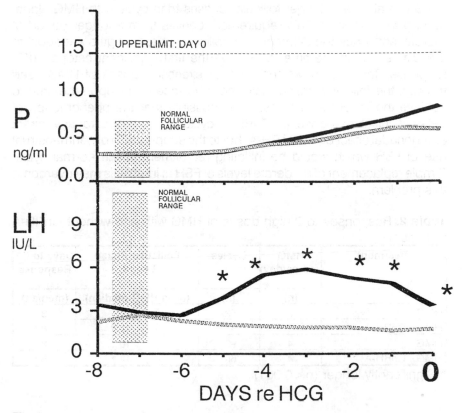

Fig. 5.
P and LH profiles of 2 series of patients undergoing OR after treatment with HMG (solid line) and with GnRH-A/HMG combined therapy (hatched line). All patients with P > 1.5 ng/ml were discontinued (HMG treatment only) and there was no difference in the P concentrations between the 2 groups. The LH showed highly significant differences (*; p < 0.001) between the groups.

nued), the LH was significantly lower in the GnRH-A cycles. There was no difference in the performance of the oocytes retrieved from these cycles suggesting that LH lowered to this degree is not essential.

Ovarian Responses

Analyses of the influence of simultaneous GnRH-A therapy upon follicular growth dynamics have shown that they are unable to influence the number recruited or the speed of growth after recruitment in PCO patients (Fleming et al, 1990) and in normal patients (Fleming and Coutts, 1986). However, it is now well established that long course therapies require more HMG overall due to longer follicular phases than cycle with HMG alone, as shown in Table 2. This requirement derives from a longer period of recruitment, since the differences in follicular phase lengths are equal to the differences in the time to achieve the first significant estogen (E2) response. Table 2, shows that high or excessive doses of HMG used through the follicular phase make no difference to, or upon the time to achieve the initial E2 response. It is possible that the phenomenon of delayed initial response in GnRH-A cycles is not due to any direct anti-gonadal effect of the GnRH-A, but to the suppression of perimenstrual rise of FSH which would be initiating recruitment in the normal cycle. Simple replacement of moderate levels of FSH at luteolysis may overcome this problem.

Table 2. Responses to 2 high doses of HMG with and without GnRH-A treatment.

Treatment	HMG (amps/day)	Cycles	Follicular Phase Length	Days to E2 Response
	(n)	(n)	(days HMG:median)	(median)
HMG	3	52	9	3
HMG + GnRH-A	3	134	12 *	6 *
HMG	4	90	10	3
HMG + GnRH-A	4	60	12 *	6 *

* Significantly longer (p < 0.001)

Short Course GnRH-A Therapy

Ideally, short course cycles should simplify the procedures for the clinician and the patient, and use the initial agonistic "flare" effect to recruit the cohort of follicles and thereby reduce the amount of HMG required while providing the benefits of the long course therapies. Figure 6 shows the hormone profiles of a single patient treated with the GnRH-A starting on cycle day 3 with the HMG on cycle day 6 and a successful pregnancy

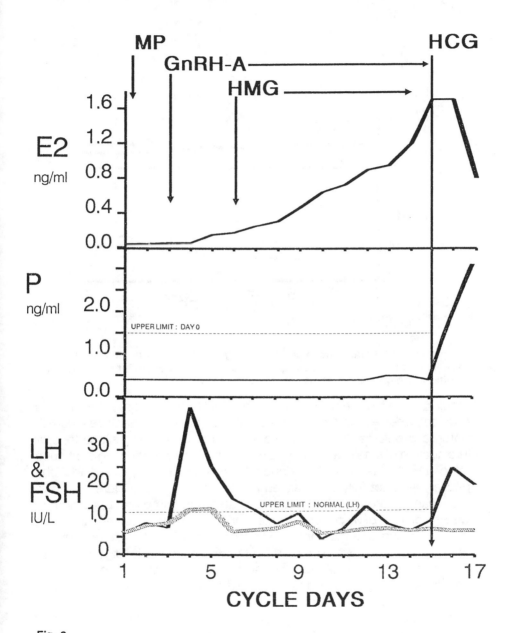

Fig. 6.
Hormone profiles of a patient undergoing a short course GnRH-A therapy with
GnRH-A starting on cycle-day 3, and the HMG starting on cycle-day 6.

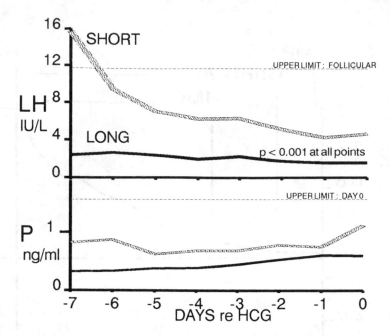

Fig. 7.
Comparison of LH and P mean profiles in long (solid line; n = 35) and short course (hatched line; n = 14) GnRH-A protocols. The concentrations of LH were significantly higher in the short course patients at all points.

resulting from a cycle with negligible pre-HCG luteinisation. However, this protocol, when applied to a series of patients revealed variable results with potential problems deriving from apparent corpus luteum rescue (and/or luteinization of small follicles), and even some patients showing continued minor LH fluctuations. The concentrations of LH suggested that the pituitary was not fully suppressed by the time of HCG. Figure 7. shows the mean LH profiles of 13 patients treated with this protocol compared with the profiles of 35 patients treated with the long protocol, and the short protocol group failed to show the 'idealised' profiles of those patients on the long course above. The result of this was increased mean P concentrations through the follicular phase at a time when the endometrium should be proliferating and not exposed to progestational influences. In some individual cases with higher than the mean P levels, this may give rise for concern, and one large series of patients treated with a similar short course (Neveu et al, 1987) showed reduced success rates compared with the long course protocol, possibly partly explained by these imperfect hormone profiles. However, improved pregnancy rates and reduced cancellation rates have been recorded, (Frydman et al, 1988) particularly in comparison with traditional treatment methods. The consumption of HMG with a short course GnRH-A applications is reduced in the normally responding patient in comparison with long course protocols. This is important where drug costs are a priority.

The Ultrashort or Sequential Protocols

Recent work investigating 'ultrashort' or sequential GnRH-A therapies in which a short period of GnRH-A therapy is given only at the start of the cycle, followed by daily HMG alone has been reported using subcutaneous GnRH-A administration (Macnamee et al, 1989). The initial data suggest that depletion of the pituitary at this time may allow follicular development without LH surge intervention. However, the mechanism for this is unclear since some cycles in the short course profiles discussed above showed undesirable LH activity during the late follicular phase, and intranasal administration in a sequential protocol still showed a high cancellation rate (Sharma et al, 1988). If intensive monitoring of LH and/or P is required in these cycles, then one of the main advantages of GnRH-A therapy is lost, and simple HMG or CC + HMG may be equally effective.

The Degree Of LH Suppression

There is some discrepancy over the duration of GnRH-A treatment required to eliminate responses to native GnRH, and the correlation of this period with reliable suppression of LH interference. The time when the pituitary is unable to respond to endogenous E2 with a positive feedback surge is probably the most important marker, and this may not be directly related to any clinical tests used.

It can be seen in Figure 5 that using the long course protocol, suppression of LH in the late follicular phase is effective to concentrations approaching the limits of assay senstivity. However, the profiles of LH seen with the short courses do not show such invariable and profound suppression, and certainly are elevated in the early stages of follicular development (day-7). In terms of influence upon follicular metabolism - luteinization at the later stages of follicular growth - this difference may be unimportant, since the concentrations recorded are within the normal range and declining, and LH surges are effectively eliminated. There appears to be no detrimental effect upon fertilization or embryo development rates amongst these cycles, so paranoia about follicular phase LH concentrations (except for +ve feedback surges) should be avoided.

Programming with GnRH-As

It is possible to plan ahead with short course GnRH-A cycles, and simulataneously avoid the risk of corpus luteum rescue or luteinization of small follicles; and thereby obviate monitoring for adverse LH activity. Pretreatment with a progestogen is followed by a menstrual bleed where-upon the GnRH-A can be initiated. This may initiate follicular recruitment and stimulation of follicular growth which is maintained by HMG adminis-tration started 3 days later (Zom et al, 1987). The desired suppression of LH during the late follicular phase appears to be achieved without any of the problems deriving from the "flare" effect upon normally stimulated ovaries.

Influence Of LH Suppression upon Embryology

The different treatments, and thereby the different hormonal environ-ments, probably affect intrafollicular metabolism and should therefore influence surgical and embryological procedures to some degree. Sup-pression of LH prior to HCG administration blocks pre-HCG luteinization and also the minor fluctuations of LH occurring by normal diurnal rhythm and/or pulsatility, and these may influence the timing of responses to the HCG or the endogenous LH surge. Most centres carry out oocyte retrieval (OR) between 32 and 36h after HCG because of data obtained from Clomid and Clomid + HMG treated cycles (Trounson et al, 1982) showing high variation in the incidence of pre-operative ovulation in cycles with luteinization to oocyte retrieval delays (LORDs) greater than 35h. Edwards and co-workers (1984) declared that pre-operative ovulation occurred rarely before 36h, so the LORD of < 36h is a compromise between relative oocyte immaturity (requiring final stages of maturation in vitro) and avoidance of pre-operative ovulation. This compromised LORD results in a requirement for pre-insemination oocyte maturation in vitro to reduce the incidence of polyspermy (Trounson et al, 1982). The use of long course GnRH-A combined therapy suppresses the LH concentrations, and probably reduces the variation in responses to the HCG. Table 3. shows that under these circumstances no ovulation was seen with a LORD of less than 39.5h indicating that a longer in vivo period of maturation is possible, and the proportion of fully expanded cumulus cell complexes was significantly increased in the groups with the longer LORDs.

Table 3. Data from patients treated with different LORDs with laparoscopic oocyte retrieval.

LORD Group	Patients	Oocyte Yield	Collapsed Follicle Seen	Mature Oocytes	Embryos Cleaved
(h)	(n)	(mean)	(n)	(%)	(%)
32 - 36	23	8.9	0	48	68
37 - 42	41	9.1	4 #	68 *	85 *

* Significant (p < 0.01)
\# No case with collapsed follicle seen before 39 1/2 h.

This apparent benefit was reflected in higher fertilization and cleavage rates in the groups with the longer in vivo maturation (LORD) times. This reduction in the biological variation of follicular and oocyte responses to therapy caused by follicular phase LH suppression may prove to be a further benefit of combined therapy not previously considered. It may allow simplification of embryological procedures such as omitting the in vitro maturation altogether (as in GIFT cycles), thus reducing oocyte manipulations at a time of high vulnerability. It has yet to be tested whether these responses are similar with short course cycles.

Problem Patients

There are sub-groups of IVF/GIFT patients who may benefit from one particular therapy in preference to another. Older patients (> 38y) do not respond at all well to Clomid in that they tend to produce relatively few follicles, with reduced plasma E2 concentrations and yield few oocytes. Using the combined therapy, these patients tend to require even more HMG, but do respond with a greater yield of oocytes and embryos (Rutherford et al, 1988). "Poor responders" is a term frequently applied to another sub-group of patients treated with Clomid + HMG who either fail to undergo OR, or produce few follicles and oocytes after protracted cycles which have a poor pregnancy potential. Some centres restrict the use of GnRH-A combined therapies to these patients, since better pregnancy results have been well demonstrated in this sub-group (Serafini et al, 1988). However, there is a significant group of patients who are poor responders on the combined therapies also. Patients with PCO are another sub-group who tend to be difficult to treat with IVF/GIFT procedures, possibly because of high basal LH, or a high frequency of LH surges. They also have a tendency to over-respond and hyperstimulate. The combined GnRH-A therapy (long course) shows clear advantages due to the suppression of LH throughout the treatment course, although the tendency to hyperstimulate is unaffected by the suppression of LH and must be guarded against by careful monitoring of the degree of response.

Summary

The highly potent GnRH-As have established a role in gynaecology through their highly effective suppression of gonadotrophin secretion and gonadal function. They suppress LH to a greater degree than FSH, and this function has been exploited during the induction of multiple follicular growth for assisted conception programmes, because of the spontaneous interference of LH in follicular development. It is well established that the LH surge (attenuated or not) interferes with the clinical manipulations of induced follicular growth, and that the GnRH-As are highly effective at blocking this effect.

It may be that high LH concentrations alone can interfere with oocyte viability, although this has yet to be proven. Long course GnRH-A cycles demonstrate LH concentrations significantly lower than either those seen in short courses or in well controlled HMG cycles without pre-HCG luteinization, and there is no difference in the performance of oocytes from any of these groups; suggesting that normal range LH concentrations do not interfere with oocyte viability. Furthermore, the dynamics of follicular growth, once established appear to be unaffected by the different levels of LH activity seen in the different types of GnRH-A or HMG alone programmes.

The low concentrations and low variability of LH in long course cycles allows longer and perhaps more precise in vivo maturation periods between HCG and OR which may prove to be a further benefit of combined therapy.

The main criticism of GnRH-A combined therapies is the increased requirement for costly HMG, but the reduced cycle cancellation rate and reduced monitoring requirements go some way to offset these extra costs. Short course therapies also may reduce drug costs somewhat, but problems of corpus luteum rescue and fluctuating LH in some circumstances remain to be studied in the different varieties available. The programmed short courses may show the greater potential in this regard although the savings in HMG may be less than hoped for in these protocols.

References

D. Mouzon J., Piette, C., & Bachelot A. (1988). Decreased fertility in relation to women's age: findings from in vitro fertilization. J. Reprod. Fert. Abstract Series. 2: No 33.

Edwards RG., Fishel, SB., Cohen J. (1984). Factors influencing the success of in vitro fertilisation for alleviating human infertility. J. In Vitro Fert and Embryo Transfer, 1. 3-23.

Edwards R.G., & Steptoe PC. (1975). Induction of follicular growth, ovulation and luteinization in the human ovary. J. Reprod. Fertil. Sup 22, 121-163.

Fleming R., Adams AH., Barlow DH., Black WP., Macnaughton MC., and Coutts JRT. (1982). A new systematic treatment for infertile women with abnormal hormone profiles. Brit. J. Obstet, Gynaecol., 80, 80-83.

Fleming R., & Coutts JRT. (1986). Induction of multiple follicular growth in normally menstruating women with endogenous gonadotropi n suppression. Fertil. Steril., 41, 827-832.

Fleming R., Hamilton MPR, Conaghan C., Black WP., & Coutts JRT. (1990). Ovarian sensitivity to gonadotrophins in patients with PCO is unaffected by suppression of LH. Clinical Endocrinology, 32, 33-38.

Frydman R., Belaisch-Allart J., Parneix, I., Forman, R., Hazout A., & Testart J. (1988). Comparison between flare-up and down regulation effects of luteinizing hormone-releasing hormone agonists in an in vitro fertilization program. Fertil. Steril. 50, 471-475.

Gougeon A., & Lefebre B. (1983). Evolution of the largest healthy and atretic follicles during the human menstrual cycle. J. Reprod Fertil, 69, 497-502.

Hackeloer BJ., Fleming R., Robinson HP, Adams AH., & Coutts JRT. (1979). Correlation of ultrasonic and endocrinological assessment of follicular development. Am J. Obstet & Gynecol., 135, 122-128.

Hillier SG., Afnan AMM., Margara RA., & Winston RML. (1985) Superovulation strategy before in vitro fertilization. Clinics in Obstet & Gynaecol, 12, 687-723.

Howles CM, Macnamee MC, Edwards RG., Goswamy, & Steptoe PC. (1986). Effects of high tonic levels of LH on outcome of In-Vitro Fertilization. Lancet ii, 521-522.

Jamieson ME., Carter ME., Hamilton MPR, Fleming R. and Coutts JRT. (1988). Oocyte Selection for GIFT - Lessons from IVF. Hum Reprod, Abstract No. 173; 53.

Messinis IE., Templeton A., & Baird DT. (1986). Relationships between the characteristics of endogenous luteinizing hormone surge and the degree of ovarian hyperstimulation during superovulation induction in women. Clin. Endocrinol. 25, 393-400.

Neveu S., Hedon B., Bringer J., Chinchole J-M, Arnal F., Humeau C., Cristol P., & Viala JL. (1987). Ovarian stimulation by a combination of a gonadotrophin releasing hormone agonist and gonadotropins for in vitro fertilization. Fertil. Steril., 47, 639-644.

Rutherford AJ., Suback-Sharpe RJ, Dawson KJ, Margara RA., Franks S., & Winston RML. (1988). Improvement of in vitro fertilisation after treatment with buserelin, an agonist of luteinising hormone releasing hormone. Brit. Med J. 296, 1765-1768.

Serafini P., Stone B., Kerin J., Batzofin J., Quin P., & Marrs RP. (1988). An alternate approach to controlled ovarian hyperstimulation in "poor responders" pretreatment with a gonadotropinreleasing hormone analog. Fertil. Steril. 49, 90-95.

Sharma V., Williams J., Collins W., Riddle A., Mason B., & Whitehead M. (1988). The sequential use of a Luteinizing Hormone-Releasing Hormone (LH-RH) agonist and human menopausal gonadotropins to stimulate folliculogenesis in women with resistant ovaries. J. In Vitro Fert. Embryo Transfer. 5, 38-42.

Stanger JD. & Yovich JL. (1985). Reduced in-vitro fertilization of human oocytes from patients with raised basal luteinizing hormone levels during the follicular phase. Brit. J. Obstet. & Gynaecol. 92, 385-393.

Thomas A., Okamoto S., O'Shae F., Maclachlan V., Besanko M. & Healey D. (1989). Do raised serum luteinizing hormone levels during sitmulation for in-vitro fertilization predict outcome? Brit. J. Obstet. Gynaecol., 96, 1328-1332.

Trounson AO., Mohr LR. Wood C., & Leeton JF. (1982). Effect of delayed insemination on in vitro fertlization, culture and transfer of human embryos. J. Reprod. Fert. 64, 285-294.

Zorn JR., Boyer P., & Guichard A. (1987). Never on a Sunday. Lancet, ii, 385.

INCLUSION OF HUMAN GROWTH HORMONE (hGH) IN STIMULATION REGIMENS FOR POOR RESPONDERS

Regulation of Follicle Growth

Superovulation is not achieved in all women despite the use of increasing amounts of human menopausal gonadotrophin (hMG). Some patients, namely "poor responders", are resistant to such a treatment. Attempts to improve the ovarian response to exogenous gonadotrophins by increasing the dose of hMG (Benadiva et al, 1988) or using GnRH analogues (Serafini et al, 1988) were met with limited success. Growth hormone has been shown to improve the ovarian response to exogenous gonadotrophins in women treated for in vivo as well as in vitro fertilization (Homburg et al, 1988).

Although the central role of gonadotrophins in the regulation of granulosa cell ontogeny is well established, the variable fate of ovarian follicles subjected to comparable gonadotrophic stimulation suggests the existence of additional intraovarian modulatory mechanisms (Adashi et al 1984). In this connection the role of several growth factors have been the subject of intense investigation.

Recent evidence suggests an important role for growth hormone and insulin like growth factor I (IGF-I) in the regulation of granulosa cell function (Adashi et al, 1984). Among potential modulators of granulosa cell ontogeny, the insulin like growth factors (IGFs) appear uniquely suited to the task, combining replicative and in some instances cytodifferentiative properties (Adashi et al, 1985).

Growth hormone (GH) is a polypeptide with a molecular weight of around 21,500 Daltons with two main actions: stimulation of general tissue growth and control of body metabolism. It is synthesised and secreted by the somatotroph cells of the anterior pituitary gland. GH is released in an episodic, pulsatile manner throughout the day, but most is released at night during periods of stage 3/4 sleep. GH is also released in various stressful conditions and by exercise, but circulating levels are largely influenced by the metabolic status of the individual.

The IGF's constitute a family of homologous, low molecular weight, single chain polypeptide growth factors, named for their remarkable structural and functional similarity to insulin (Zapf et al 1981). Whereas insulin may have assumed the responsibility for the maintenance of homeostasis in fuel economy (King & Kahn 1981), the IGFs together with other factors, appear concerned with the initiation and maintenance of mesenchymal tissue growth (Bradshaw & Sporn 1982).

Growth hormone stimulates general tissue growth through the mediation of IGF-I (formerly known as Somatomedin-C), large amounts of which are produced in the liver (Phillips and Vassipoulou 1978). Somatomedin-C/IGF-I displays stringent growth hormone (GH) dependence in vivo and in vitro (Adashi et al 1985). However IGF-I is also produced in a wide variety of tissues, where it may be active in a paracrine rather than an endocrine manner (D'Ercole et al 1984).

Growth Hormone and Ovarian Function

In 1972 Sheikholism and Stempfel demonstrated that delayed puberty associated with isolated GH deficiency is readvanced by GH therapy. GH administered to hypophysectomised female rats increases the in vitro steroidogenic responsiveness to gonadotrophins (Advis et al, 1981). Intraovarian peptides were suggested to play a role in local control of follicular development (Hammond 1981). In particular, IGF-I has been shown to synergize with FSH in the induction of rat granulosa cell aromatase activity (Adashi et al, 1985), with increased level of oestrogen, progesterone, and number and binding capabity of LH receptors. This ability of IGF-I to potentiate FSH driven ovarian functions (Jia et al, 1986) may account at least in part for the puberty promoting effect of growth hormone. Growth hormone has also been shown to increase the ovarian level of IGF-I in vivo in the rat (Davoren and Hsueh, 1986) suggesting that growth hormone may affect ovarian differentiation by inducing the local production or accumulation of IGF-I, and providing evidence for a novel intraovarian paracrine control mechanism.

The GH dependent generation of intraovarian IGF-I, and the consequent local potentiation of gonadotrophin dependent ovarian function in rats, initiated studies in women with ovaries previously shown to be resistent to gonadotrophin. The first report came from Homburg et al in 1988. They treated four patients by in vivo and three patients by in vitro fertilization, all previously resistant to treatment with hMG. These patients received biosynthetic human growth hormone (B-hGH; Norditropin, Nordisk Gentofte, A/S) 20 IU on alternate days for 2 weeks in combination with hMG. This concomitant treatment with B-hGH and hMG showed augmented ovarian response in all treated patients with a decrease in mean number of treatment days and number of hMG ampoules needed. In the IVF patients, an increased number of oocytes were collected. Three patients conceived, one by in vivo and two by in vitro fertilization. These data offered a new approach to stimulation of ovarian function by utilising known endocrine effects to influence paracrine control of ovarian function.

Studies Using Biosynthetic Human Growth Hormone

In the IVF unit at St Mary's Hospital, Manchester, we wanted to investigate further the effect of B-hGH on the ovarian response when administered in combination with hMG or hMG and buserelin to patients undergoing IVF and being previously poor responders to conventional treatment for induction of ovulation. We carried out three pilot studies using three different regimes of ovulation induction in combination with B-hGH (Norditropin, Nordisk Gentofte, A/S). The criteria for inclusion in the studies were:

1. Previously poor responders to treatment for induction of ovulation, i.e. in need of 3 or more ampoules of hMG per day, having reduced production of oestrogen and/or reduced number of follicles > 14 mm.
2. < 40 years old.
3. Normal basal gonadotrophins (FSH < 10 IU/L).
4. No evidence of hypertension, diabetes mellitus or impaired glucose tolerance.
5. Normal prolactin level.

STUDY 1:

Five patients previously poor responders to treatment with clomiphene citrate and hMG for induction of ovulation were studied. They received a combined treatment of hMG (in the same previous daily dose) and B-hGH (24 IU on alternate days for a maximum of 6 injections) for one cycle. Both hMG and B-hGH started on day 3 of the cycle. In all five patients the previous cycle was cancelled due to poor response. In the study cycles only 2 cycles were cancelled due to poor response. One patient ovulated spontaneously before oocyte recovery and the cycle was abandoned.

In the two patients who reached oocyte recovery, a mean of 3 eggs were recovered and a mean of 2 embryos were replaced. One patient became pregnant following embryo replacement, and has delivered a healthy baby at term.

Four of the 5 GH cycles showed a spontaneous LH surge. There were however no serious side effects noted with the GH treatment.

In this small group of patients the use of GH in conjunction with hMG for ovulation induction did not result in any significant improvement in the ovarian response either in the number of follicles recruited or in the oestradiol levels over the previous stimulation regime of CC/hMG.

In a similar study, Volpe et al (1989) treated 12 low responding patients with a combination of GH and gonadotrophins (hMG and FSH). All patients, aged 26-41, had proved resistant to gonadotrophin therapy. They observed a low ovarian response in all 4 patients above 40 years of age. A satisfactory ovarian response was however detected in all 8 younger patients (<35 years) with better follicular recruitment. However no clinical pregnancy was achieved.

STUDY II:

Five patients previously poor responders to an ultra short course of buserelin (500 ug/day from day 2-4 of the cycle) and hMG were investigated. They received the same day regime of buserelin and hMG together with B-hGH (24 IU on alternate days for a maximum of 6 injections) starting with the hMG on day 3 of the cycle.

While 3 of the previous cycles were cancelled due to poor response, only one of the GH cycles was cancelled. Four patients reached the stage of oocyte recovery as compared to only 2 in their previous cycles. Oocytes were recovered from only 2 of these 4 patients. Two embryos were replaced in 2 patients, but no pregnancy was achieved. One important observation however was the occurence of an LH surge in 3 of the 5 GH cycles and a start of LH rise in a fourth cycle. This observation was only made when GH was added to the ultrashort course of buserelin and hMG and raises the possibility of an enhancing effect of GH on the positive feedback mechanism which initiates the LH surge.

The use of B-hGH in conjunction with an ultrashort term buserelin regime and hMG did not result in any improvement in the ovarian response or IVF outcome. These results were substantiated by the results of the Finnish group from the University of Oulu (Ronnberg et al 1989). They treated 38 women by IVF in a placebo double blind controlled study using a short course of intrasal buserelin (600 ug/day 1-4), with hMG in addition to B-hGH or placebo. They failed to show any advantage from the addition of B-hGH to their stimulation regime, either in the dose of hMG or the length of treatment. Similarly no difference in oestradiol or progesterone production in the follicular phase was found between the GH or the placebo group. There was also no difference in the number of follicles, number of oocytes, cleavage or fertilization rate between the 2 groups.

STUDY III:

The results of our first two pilot studies using B-hGH in conjunction with hMG or ultra short term buserelin regime and hMG were not encouraging. No significant benefit was shown from the addition of B-hGH to conventional stimulation regimes in poor responders. No more follicles were recruited and no improvement in serum oestradiol was demonstrated. The control of the cycles was difficult as many patients demonstrated premature LH surges which led either to abandoning the cycle if there was no more than 1 follicle present or proceeding to oocyte recovery with premature follicles.

We therefore recruited 10 more patients who have shown a poor response to a long term buserelin regime (starting in the midluteal phase) and hMG (Matson et al 1989). Poor response was defined as the need for 4 or more ampoules (>300 IU) of hMG per day. All ten patients however reached oocyte recovery in their previous cycle.

They received the same buserelin/hMG regime together with B-hGH starting with the hMG. Five patients received 12 IU/day for 12 injections, and 5 patients received 24 IU on alternate days for 6 injections. The same criteria for hCG administration were applied as in the previous cycle i.e. 3 follicles of 20 mm or more. A further injection of hCG 2,000 IU was given in all cycles as a luteal support 4 days post-oocyte recovery.

The results of the study are shown in Table 1. As there was no statistical difference between the results of the two growth hormone regimens, the results were combined.

The use of human growth hormone in conjuction with long term buserelin regime has significantly reduced the length of the "follicular phase" of the treatment cycle i.e. the number of days of hMG administration with a concomitant decrease in the total number of ampoules of hMG needed per cycle. This shortening of the follicular phase was due to a significant increase in the rate of follicular growth per day.

However the number of follicles >14mm on the day of the ovulatory trigger and the serum oestradiol concentration on that day, were not increased by the inclusion of growth hormone in the stimulation regimen. A further effect noticed was the increased number of oocytes collected in the treatment cycles using growth hormone which resulted in an in-

Table 1 Results of the treatment cycles in study III using buserelin/hMG or buserelin/hMG/growth hormone [mean(sd)].

Parameter	buserelin/hMG (n = 10)	buserelin/hMG/GH (n = 10)
days of hMG	19.6 (3.56)	14.6 (2.91) ***
hMG/cycle (amps.)	91.8 (34.9)	58.8 (18.9) **
foll. growth/day (mm)	1.28 (0.42)	1.74 (0.47) *
no. folls. >14mm #	5.5 (2.4)	6.3 (2.7)
serum oestradiol (pg/ml)	1461 (644)	1318 (641)
oocytes collected	4.1 (3.1)	7.2 (3.6) ***
embryos replaced (n = 8)	1.25 (1.39)	2.6 (0.75) *
no. of replacements	4 (+1 GIFT)	10
no. pregnancies	0	6

   \# on day of hCG
   * $p < 0.05$, ** $p < 0.01$, *** $p < 0.001$

creased number of embryos replaced in the IVF cycles (excluding one patient who had previously been treated by GIFT and another in whom no oocytes had been collected in the first cycle). Interestingly 6 out of the 10 women conceived in their growth hormone cycle (5 singleton and one twin). All six women have already delivered healthy babies.

In this study a state of hypogonadotrophic hypogonadism was achieved (medical hypophysectomy) before administration of hMG and B-hGH. This is probably of importance and is consistent with the results of Homburg et al (1988), and Blumenfeld and Lunenfeld (1989), who treated women with hypogonadotrophic hypogonadism.

Blumenfeld and Lunenfeld (1989) treated one patient with panyhypopituitarism with combined hMG and B-hGH and she conceived on her 2nd cycle of this regime. In a state of hypogonadotrophic hypogonadism GH is administered when the ovaries are quiescent and follicular recruitment by exogenous gonadotrophin is just beginning. This may be the time the follicles are most in need of a growth promoting factor. Another possible explanation for the favourable ovarian response to this regime is that the very low levels of endogenous gonadotrophins, either in hypogonadotrophic hypogonadism or after the administration of GnRH analogues, may render the ovaries more sensitive to action of GH. This study has clearly demonstrated an enhancement by growth hormone of the rate of follicular growth if not the number of follicles recruited. The pregnancy rate achieved in this small sample is very encouraging. As there was no difference in the peak oestradiol nor the number of follicles >14 mm recruited on the day of hCG, this favourable outcome cannot be attributed solely to improved folliculogenesis but may reflect the increased number of preovulatory oocytes collected and possibly enhanced endometrial receptivity. While the total amount of hMG used was reduced by a third, this cost reduction is still outweighed by the cost of the additional course of B-hGH used. However, if the pregnancy rate obtained in this small sample of patients is sustained the drug cost may be justified especially in a group of patients whose prognosis was otherwise very poor.

IGF-I was assessed pretreatment as well as 5 days after the start of B-hGH (12 hours after the last GH injection). This showed a rise in 9 of the 10 patients over a basal level of IGF-I, suggesting an action of GH in increasing serum IGF-I. However the rise in IGF-I was not significantly different between those patients who achieved a pregnancy and those who did not, suggesting that the level of IGF-I acheived following GH treatment may be of poor prognostic value for the establishment of a pregnancy.

There was however a higher increase in IGF-I in patients receiving daily injections of GH than in patients receiving alternate days injection. This may be related to the higher pregnancy rate achieved in the first group (4 out of 5) than in the second group (2 out of 5).

Future Studies

Further prospective studies are now needed to confirm the preliminary data obtained in Study III. Prospective studies are also needed in order to:

1. Establish the minimal effective dose of B-hGH required to produce an optimum ovarian response.
2. Determine the optimum length of time B-hGH treatment is required in the follicular phase.
3. Investigate the effect of B-hGH on the endometrium.
4. Evaluate the role of GH in "normal responders."

If a similar or better pregnancy rate can be achieved in "normal responders" GH treatment may in future become an essential element in the treatment of infertile couples.

References

Adashi, E.Y., Resnick, C.E., Svoboda, M.E. & Van Wyk, J.J. (1984). A novel role for sonatomedin-C in the cytodifferentiation of the ovarian granulosa cells. Endocrinology, 115: 1227-1229.

Adashi, E.Y., Resnick, C.E., d'Ercole, A.J., Svoboda, M.E. & Van Wyk, J.J. (1985). Insulin-like growth factors as intraovarian regulators of granulosa cell growth and function. Endocrine reviews 6 : 400-420

Advis, J.P., Smith White, S. & Ojeda, S.R. (1981). Activation of growth hormone short loop negative feedback delays puberty in the female rat. Endocrinology, 108: 1343.

Benadiva, C.A., Ben Rafael, Z., Strauss, J.F., Mastorianni, L., Flickinger, G.L. (1988). Ovarian response of individuals to different doses of human menopausal gonadotrophin. Fertil Steril. 49: 997-1001.

Blumenfeld, Z. and Lunenfeld, B. (1989). The potentiating effect of growth hormone on follicle stimulation with human menopausal gonadotrophin in a panhypopituitary patient. Fertil Steril. 52: 328-331.

Davoren, J.B. and Hsueh, A.J.W. (1986). Growth hormone increases ovarian levels of immuno reactive somatomedin C/insulin like growth factor I in vivo. Endocrinology 118, 888-890.

D'Ercole, A.J., Stiles, A.D., & Underwood, L.E. (1984). Tissue concentrations of somatomedin C: Further evidence for multiple sites of synthesis and paracrine or autocrine mechanism of action. Proc. Natl. Acad. Sci. USA 81: 935-939.

Hammond, J.M. (1981) Peptide regulators in the ovarian follicle. Aust J Biol Sciences, 34, 491-504.

Homburg, R., Eshel, A., Abdalla, H.I., Jacobs, H.S. (1988) Growth hormone facilitates ovulation induction by gonadotrophins. Clin. Endocrinol. 29: 113-117.

Jia, X.C., Kalmijn, J., Hsueh, A.J.W. (1986). Growth hormone enhances follicle-stimulating hormone-induced differentiation of cultured rat granulosa cells. Endocrinology 118: 1401-1409.

King, G.L. and Kahn, C.R. (1981). Non parallel evolution of metabolic and growth promoting functions of insulin. Nature 292: 644.

Matson, P., Ibrahim, Z., Buck, P., Burslem R.W., Isherwood, P., and Lieberman, B.A. (1989). Human in-vitro fertilisation and embryo transfer following pituitary down regulation with buserelin. J Endocrinol 121: supplement, 306.

Phillips, L.S. and Vassilopoulou - Sellin R (1980). Somatomedins. New Eng. J. Med. 302: 371-380.

Serafini, P., Stone, B., Kerin, J., Batzofin, J., Quinn, P., Marrs, R.P., (1988). An alternate approach to controlled ovarian hyperstimulation in "poor responders": pretreatment with a gonadotrophin-releasing hormone analog. Fertil Steril 49: 90-96.

Ronnberg, L., Tapanainen, J., Martikainen, H., Puistola, U., and Orava, M. (1989). Use of growth hormone in hyperstimulation for in vitro fertilisation. Presented at the 5th annual meeting of the European Society of Human Reproduction and Embryology. Malmo. Abstract M9:4

Sheikholislam, B.M. and Stempfel, R.S. (1972). Hereditary isolated somatoropin deficiency: effects of human growth hormone administration. Paediatrics 49: 362-374.

Volpe A., Minuto F., Barreca A., Coukos G., Artini PG., Silferi M., Genazzani R., (1989). Combined growth hormone plus gonadotrophins for induction of superovulation in hypogonadotrophic and low responding patients. Presented at the XIII world congress on Fertility and Sterility, Marrakesh. Abstract No. 309.

Zapf, J., Froesch, E., Humbel, R.E., (1981). The insulin like growth factors (IGF) of human serum: Chemical and biological characterization and aspects of their possible physiological role. Curr Top Cell Reg 19: 257.

3   S. Fishel, S. Antinori, J. Webster

EVALUATION OF THE INCLUSION OF FSH IN FOLLICULAR STIMULATION REGIMES

Introduction

Various hormonal preparations for the stimulation of follicular growth in anovulatory and oligo- and amenorrhoeic females have been used for nearly 30 years. Since the advent of in vitro fertilization (IVF) and associated techniques, a range of follicular stimulation regimes have been used on the normal cyclical female (Fishel and Jackson, 1989).

There are three principle reasons why follicular stimulation became engraved in IVF treatment. First, fewer patients were cancelled during the follicular phase as a result of the difficulty of monitoring the LH surge. Second, and probably the most important principle, was the observation that there was a significant increase in the incidence of pregnancy when the numbers of conceptuses replaced increased from 1 to 3, ie. from 10-15% for the replacement of 1 conceptus to over 40% for the replacement of 3 conceptuses (Fishel and Jackson, 1989). It was also demonstrated that by giving follicular stimulants more patients received 2 and 3 conceptuses than in natural cycles where over 95% patients received 1 conceptus (Fishel et al, 1985). Thirdly, follicular stimulation was eventually shown to have the further advantage of controlling endogenous LH secretion and particularly the LH surge. The LH surge is triggered by the dominant follicle, and at this stage the dominat follicle has induced inhibitory effects on follicles in the ipsilateral and contralateral ovary resulting in fewer "fertilizable" oocytes, the spontaneous LH surge often occurred outside normal hours creating difficulties for oocyte recovery, and patients who have a high tonic LH do not respond as well to treatment, and this could often be overcome by the administration of follicular stimulants.

Follicular stimulation can recruit a large cohort of follicles from the growing pool and continued gonadotrophin support is necessary to

rescue follicles otherwise destined to atresia. Historically, follicular stimulation first succeeded using clomiphene citrate, and subsequently a
combination of clomiphene citrate and human menopausal gonadotrophin (Pergonal; Serono Laboratories). More recently, the use of FSH
(Metrodin; Serono Laboratories) alone or in conjunction with Pergonal has
been successfully employed by many units world-wide. The introduction
of gonadotrophins such as Pergonal and Metrodin circumvent the action
of the hypothalamus and pituitary as they act directly upon ovarian tissue
in a more non-physiological manner than, for example, clomiphene citrate.
Bolus injections by-pass the natural pulsatile release of these gonadotrophins which normally display specific frequency and amplitude of secretion.

When assessing data for follicular stimulation on IVF, it is necessary to
sub-group patients in order to evaluate their response. For example, 3
main types of patients may be identified, (i) those poor or low responders
- judged either by the lack of numerous follicles stimulated or the quality
of the oestradiol-17B (E_2) pattern - but with otherwise normal endocrinology, (ii) those patients who have high tonic LH, especially with the LH:FSH
ratios outside the normal range during the early and late follicular phase,
and (iii) those patients who in every respect appear endocrinologically
normal. Early FSH enrichment via exogenous Metrodin has been tried by
many groups in all types of patients, and the beneficial nature of Metrodin
is still being evaluated.

A number of studies, including the early work of Jones et al (1984) and
the follow-up studies of Bernadus et al (1985) superimposing Metrodin on
a Pergonal cycle had very encouraging results. In this regime, 2 ampoules
of Pergonal were given from day 3 of the cycle and 2 ampoules of Metrodin
on days 3 and 4 of the cycle only, continuing stimulation with Pergonal.
This study was done with patients who had an inadequate response on
the ordinary regime of 2 ampoules of Pergonal daily from day 3. The
results of this study demonstrated a dose-related enhancement effect of
FSH for follicular recruitment and development. The numbers of fertilized
oocytes and overall pregnancy rate when follicular enhancement was
induced with FSH was significantly higher with an overall pregnancy rate
of 28% per replacement. It is important to note that this study compared
only those patients who were poor responders on the Pergonal only
regime. The multi-centre trial by Bundren et al (1990) adopted the regime
of 150 iu's per day (2 ampoules) of Metrodin daily from day 2 of a cycle
until 2 follicles reached a diameter of approximately 16 mm. Approximately
35% of patients had cycles abandoned because of poor folllicular development, and the overall incidence of pregnancy was 24% per laparoscopy

and 60% of these went to delivery. However, it was clear from this study that there was enormous patient variation to stimulation.

In 1988, Navot and Rosenwaks published the various stimulation regimes practiced by the Norfolk group over the last 5 years. Four main groups of stimulation were described, the first 2 being combination groups of Pergonal or Metrodin. This is a regime which is not only augmenting recruitment but the addition of Metrodin is described as having a "boost" effect on selection. In addition, there were 3 Metrodin only regimes. In assessing IVF regimes it is necessary to relate all data to the "bottom line"; which we define as being able to utilise follicular stimulation regimes which will permit the maximum number of patients through to oocyte recovery and achieve the highest incidence of deliveries per treatment cycle *balanced against* the unnecessary administration of drugs, increasing costs, hyperfolliculation and hyperstimulation (for discussion see Fishel and Jackson, 1989). Table 1 describes the 4 main groups of Navot and

Table 1. 5 Years' Experience - from Navot and Rosenwaks (1988)

Regime	Gonadotrophin	Administration
COMBO 1	2 ampoules Pergonal	3 →
	2 ampoules Metrodin	3 & 4
	'Augmentation of recruitment'	
COMBO 2	2 ampoules Pergonal	3 →
	2 ampoules Metrodin	3,4,5,6
	'boosting selection and rescuing follicles from atresia'	
P-FSH REGIMES	Either 2 ampoules Metrodin	3 →
	or 3 ampoules Metrodin thereafter 2 or 3 ampoules 'enhanced recruitment and selection'	3 & 4
	or 4 ampoules Metrodin thereafter 2 ampoules 'enhanced p-FSH protocol'	3 & 4
PERGONAL ONLY	2 ampoules Pergonal	→

→ continued to ovulation induction

Rosenwaks' study which consist of 6 actual regimes. The first combination regime of Metrodin and Pergonal was described as an augmentation of recruitment, the second combination regime in which Metrodin was given for 4 days up to day 6 in combination with Pergonal from day 3 was described as a regime boosting selection and rescuing follicles from atresia. A summary of the data from these regimes is expressed in Table 2. Evaluating the data demonstrates that the "combo 1" regime had the

highest incidence of pregnancy and viable pregnancy, the shortest duration of exogenous gonadotrophins and adequate E_2 patterns. The
"combo 2" regime was described as having few good E_2 patterns. The
Metrodin only regimes had the disadvantage of requiring large amounts
of Metrodin with the regime using 2 ampoules only having the lowest
miscarriage rate, and this regime along with the Pergonal only regime had
the highest incidence of favourable E_2 patterns. According to the "bottom
line" maxim, although the data has to be based on pregnancies and
deliveries, it is clear that the best regime was the combination regime using
Pergonal 2 ampoules from day 3 and Metrodin 2 ampoules on days 3 and
4 continuing with Pergonal only to ovulation induction. This was the most
suitable regime for patients being stimulated for the first time.

Table 2. Results of Norfolk Data *

Regime	Pregnancy Rate #	Viable Preg. Rate	Miscarriage Rate	Cancellation Rate
'COMBO 1'	25.4 %	18.0 %	28.9 %	8.6 %
'COMBO 2' p-FSH	21.1 %	12.4 %	41.5 %	18.8 %
2 AMPS	17.0 %	12.2 %	28.6 %	6.8 %
3 AMPS	22.7 %	14.4 %	30.0 %	8.0 %
4 AMPS	23.3 %	16.5 %	29.8 %	6.9 %
PERGONAL ONLY	21.5 %	16.9 %	21.4 %	34.0 %

* Navot & Rosenwaks (1988)
# Per E.R.

More recently the use of GnRH agonists, such as buserelin, has
required an increase in the amount of follicular stimulation. However, the
main effect of the introduction of the superagonist buserelin has been to
drastically reduce the numbers of patients with abandoned cycles in the
follicular phase, thereby increasing the overall numbers of patients having
a delivery per treatment cycle. A number of regimes are now employed
for the administration of buserelin which includes long term administration
intra-nasally, or more shorter duration of administrations sub-cutaneously.
Using the superagonist and gonadotrophins, typically between 90-95% of
patients who were stimulated reached oocyte recovery compared with
between 50-75% in the previously mentioned regimes. Stimulation is
initiated and continued during an environment of consistently low endogenous gonadotrophin levels. A number of follicular stimulation
regimes have been tried consisting basically of Pergonal only using 2-4

ampoules daily, the 4 ampoule regime is often given as 2 ampoules bi-daily, or Pergonal combined with Metrodin such that Metrodin is given on the first day of stimulation for 2,3, or 4 days in a dose of either 1 or 2 ampoules a day and on the third day Pergonal is administered. Using this regime it is possible to boost the follicular quota depending on the number of ampoules of Metrodin that have been used.

Here we have evaluated 5 follicular stimulation regimes, 3 using buserelin where the dosage of Pergonal was varied according to the response of the patient but the administration of Metrodin was given at random as either 4 ampoules (2 ampoules on days 1 and 2) or 6 ampoules (given as 2 ampoules on days 1, 2 and 3), or without the use of Metrodin using Pergonal only with a minimum of 3 ampoules from day 2. Two further regimes were evaluated retrospectively and used simply Clomid (100 mg from days 2-6) and Pergonal (2 ampoules from day 5) or in a few patients Metrodin 2 ampoules (1 ampoule on days 1 and 2) with continued gonadotrophin stimulation from Pergonal only.

Observation And Discussion

As the older patient tends to have a reduced response to gonadotrophins compared to the younger patient, those analysed in this study were aged between 28 and 36 years of age. Of the 310 patients evaluated not all information was available or reliable from every patient and therefore only those with accurate data were assessed. When the outcome of the treatment was assessed according to the numbers of conceptuses replaced there was no significant difference in establishing implantation or delivery. With the use of buserelin there was a highly significant reduction in the incidence of cycles cancelled during the follicular phase (8.5%) compared to the Clomid and Pergonal regime of 26.5% and the Metrodin and Pergonal regime (21%). Only those patients with tubal factor or no overt male infertility factor were assessed to prevent a bias when evaluating the number of oocytes fertilized.

When buserelin was incorporated into the stimulation regime significantly more Pergonal was required for stimulation than the other 2 regimes, although the use of Metrodin significantly reduced the number of ampoules of Pergonal required for adequate follicular growth (Table 3). Without the use of buserelin, when Metrodin was used instead of clomiphene citrate (Clomid) significantly more Pergonal was also necessary (Table 3). Apart from the additional gonadotrophins required for adequate follicular growth, this generally imparts an additional cost to the patient.

Table 3. Follicular Stimulation Regimes - No. Ampoules of Pergonal.

	1 BUSERELIN /P METRODIN 4 AMPS	2 BUSERELIN /P METRODIN 6 AMPS	3 BUSERELIN /P	4 CLOMID/P	5 METRODIN /P 2 AMPS
NO.	69	69	41	69	17
X	17.1	21.3	32.1	9.5	14.4
SEM	0.7	1.5	2.7	0.3	2.0
SD	5.8	12.2	17.1	2.6	8.1
MIN	6	10	12	4	6
MAX	32	68	82	17	35

1 v 2 : $p < 0.02$ 3 v 5 : $p < 0.002$
1 v 4 : $p < 0.002$
4 v 5 : $p < 0.03$

Table 4. Follicular Stimulation Regimes - Day of Oocyte Recovery.

	1 BUSERELIN /P METRODIN 4 AMPS	2 BUSERELIN /P METRODIN 6 AMPS	3 BUSERELIN /P	4 CLOMID/P	5 METRODIN /P 2 AMPS
NO.	85	85	37	85	18
X	14.0	15.4	13.3	13.2	13.1
SEM	0.26	0.25	0.29	0.14	0.59
SD	2.36	2.31	1.77	1.32	2.52
MIN	9	12	10	11	10
MAX	21	21	17	19	20

1 v 2 : $p < 0.02$ 1 v 4 : $p < 0.006$
1 v 3 : ns $p < 0.06$
2 v 3 : $p < 0.002$

The length of the follicular phase was significantly extended in this study in those patients using buserelin when 6 ampoules of Metrodin was administered compared to 4 ampoules of Pergonal alone. There was no significant difference between using 4 ampoules of Metrodin or Pergonal alone. The incorporation of 4 ampoules of Metrodin into the buserelin regime significantly extended the follicular phase by a day over the standard clomiphene and Pergonal regime (Table. 4). The levels of E_2 are shown in Table 5. On the buserelin regime 6 ampoules of Metrodin induced a significantly higher level of E_2 than the 4 ampoule regime, but

Table 5. Follicular Stimulation Regimes - Plasma E_2 - pg/ml.

	1	2	3	4	5
	BUSERELIN /P METRODIN 4 AMPS	BUSERELIN /P METRODIN 6 AMPS	BUSERELIN /P	CLOMID/P	METRODIN /P 2 AMPS
NO.	70	70	40	70	16
X	1175	1494	1331	1430	1103
SEM	5.9	7.0	15.1	6.8	10.0
SD	49.1	58.2	95.2	56.5	40.0
MIN	40	52	13	54	57
MAX	240	260	620	290	175

1 v 2 : $p < 0.002$
1 v 4 : $p < 0.007$
4 v 5 : $p < 0.02$

Table 6. Follicular Stimulation Regimes - No. Ovulatory Follicles.

	1	2	3	4	5
	BUSERELIN /P METRODIN 4 AMPS	BUSERELIN /P METRODIN 6 AMPS	BUSERELIN /P	CLOMID/P	METRODIN /P 2 AMPS
NO.	70	70	40	70	17
X	9.51	10.74	12.57	6.04	5.88
SEM	0.65	0.64	0.79	0.33	0.75
SD	5.4	5.37	5.01	2.73	3.10
MIN	2.0	2.0	3.0	1.0	1.0
MAX	35.0	31.0	30.0	16.0	12.0

1 v 3 : $p < 0.005$ 3 v 5 : $p < 0.002$
1 v 4 : $p < 0.002$
3 v 4 : $p < 0.002$

the levels of E_2 for Clomid and Pergonal were similar to the 6 ampoule regime. These levels were significantly lower on the Metrodin and Pergonal alone regime. The relationships between the plasma E_2 levels and the numbers of ovulatory follicles are shown in Tables 6 and 7. The incorporation of Metrodin into the buserelin regime produced significantly fewer oocytes than those on the Pergonal alone, but all buserelin regimes produced significantly more oocytes than those patients on Clomid and Pergonal or Metrodin and Pergonal (Table 6). The E_2:follicle ratio was similar for the 2 buserelin regimes incorporating Metrodin but these were

Table 7. Follicular Stimulation Regimes - E_2 : Follicle.

	1	2	3	4	5
	BUSERELIN /P METRODIN 4 AMPS	BUSERELIN /P METRODIN 6 AMPS	BUSERELIN /P	CLOMID/P	METRODIN /P 2 AMPS
NO.	69	69	40	69	17
X	154.7	153.3	102.2	273.7	206.2
SEM	12.7	6.6	6.2	19.0	20.0
SD	105.4	55.2	39.3	158.1	82.4
MIN	26	77	47	92.6	94.6
MAX	750	289	267	1174	405

1 v 3 : $p < 0.002$ 4 v 5 : $p < 0.02$
2 v 3 : $p < 0.002$ 3 v 5 : $p < 0.002$
3 v 4 : $p < 0.002$

Table 8. Follicular Stimulation Regimes - No. of Oocytes.

	1	2	3	4	5
	BUSERELIN /P METRODIN 4 AMPS	BUSERELIN /P METRODIN 6 AMPS	BUSERELIN /P	CLOMID/P	METRODIN /P 2 AMPS
NO.	70	68	41	70	17
X	6.1	8.2	9.5	5.6	5.4
SEM	0.58	0.59	0.67	0.32	0.69
SD	4.8	4.9	4.3	2.7	2.8
MIN	1	3	2	1	1
MAX	23	29	21	15	11

1 v 2 : $p < 0.02$ 3 v 5 : $p < 0.002$
1 v 3 : $p < 0.02$ 2 v 5 : $p < 0.006$
3 v 4 : $p < 0.02$

significantly higher than patients on Pergonal alone. It is important to note, and it has been a principle well established with the incorporation of buserelin in follicular stimulation regimes, that the E_2:follicle ratio is significantly reduced whatever the gonadotrophin stimulation compared to follicular stimulation regimes not utilising buserelin. In this study there were significantly higher E_2:follicle ratios for the Clomid and Pergonal regime compared to the Metrodin and Pergonal regime, but both these regimes were significantly higher than the 3 buserelin regimes. The lower E_2:follicle ratio did not reflect the overall recovery of the number of "fertilizable"

Table 9. Follicular Stimulation Regimes - No. of Oocytes Fertilised.

	1 BUSERELIN /P METRODIN 4 AMPS	2 BUSERELIN /P METRODIN 6 AMPS	3 BUSERELIN /P	4 CLOMID/P	5 METRODIN /P 2 AMPS
NO.	48	55	40	66	15
X	3.3	4.6	5.8	4.4	3.7
SEM	0.36	0.36	0.45	0.29	0.44
SD	2.5	2.6	2.8	2.3	1.7
MIN	1	1	1	1	1
MAX	10	10	16	10	7

1 v 2 : $p < 0.02$ 3 v 4 : $p < 0.009$
1 v 3 : $p < 0.002$ 3 v 5 : $p < 0.003$
2 v 3 : $p < 0.04$

oocytes (Tables 8 and 9). Significantly more oocytes and more fertilized oocytes were obtained when 6 ampoules of Metrodin were used compared to 4 ampoules on the buserelin regime, but with Pergonal alone on the buserelin regime the numbers of oocytes and fertilized oocytes was significantly higher than both the Metrodin regimes. Generally, there was a significant increase in the number of oocytes and fertilized oocytes when patients were administered buserelin compared to the Clomid and Pergonal and Metrodin and Pergonal only regimes. No significant difference was seen between Clomid and Pergonal and Metrodin and Pergonal in either the number of oocytes recovered or fertilized.

The overall conclusions from this data when buserelin is incorporated into follicular stimulation regimes are:
(i) compared to the regime incorporating 4 ampoules of Metrodin, that using 6 ampoules significantly increases the amount of Pergonal required, the length of the follicular phase, the plasma E_2 and the number of fertilized oocytes. However, the outcome per cycle is not significantly different because there is no significant difference between groups in the numbers of patients (60-70%) receiving 3 or 4 conceptuses.
(ii) the use of Pergonal alone with buserelin significantly increases the amount of Pergonal required, the number of follicles and oocytes compared to the 4 ampoule of Metrodin regime, and significantly increases the number of fertilized oocytes over the Metrodin regimes. However, the length of the follicular phase is significantly decreased as is the E_2:follicle ratio. Therefore, it is possible to conclude from this analysis that the main advantage of a Metrodin "boost" is to reduce the amount of Pergonal

required for adequate follicular stimulation, and 2 ampoules on days 1 to 2 should be sufficient. This is in agreement with the recent study of Messinis and Templeton (1990) where they demonstrated that the follicles of 18 mm were reached 2 days earlier in stimulation regimes incorporating an FSH boost. These authors also demonstrated that the incorporation of Metrodin early in the follicular phase did not significantly affect the rate of follicular growth and assumed that the beneficial effect was for follicular stimulation at the recruitment-selection stage.

When Clomid and Pergonal was compared to Metrodin and Pergonal without the incorporation of buserelin, Metrodin significantly increased the amount of Pergonal required for adequate follicular stimulation but decreased the E_2: follicle ratio and plasma E_2 levels. There was no significant decrease in the length of the follicular phase, numbers of follicles, oocytes and fertilized oocytes obtained. Therefore, it is valid to conclude from the patients in this study that there were no obvious advantages of Metrodin boost if buserelin was not incorporated into the stimulation regime.

It is important to note that in this study the poor or non-responders were omitted, permitting an evaluation of normo-ovulatory women. In these patients, therefore, in summary, it can be concluded that there is no evidence to support the value of Metrodin "boosting" in normal ovulatory women, and there is no evidence to support its addition to routine stimulation regimes in terms of results. There may be a significant improvement in reducing cancellations in the follicular phase and reducing the number of ampoules of Pergonal required for adequate follicular stimulation with the use of buserelin. However, a few studies have demonstrated enhanced overall IVF success when Metrodin is superimposed on Pergonal stimulation, with or without buserelin, in difficult or non-responders. But the multi-centre trial of Bundren et al (1990), in contrast to the data of Jones et al (1985), demonstrated a cancellation rate of 35% with an overall pregnancy rate of 24% and 29.4% for those patients receiving 3 conceptuses, using Metrodin alone. The recent study of Karande et al (1990) demonstrated no significant difference in "low responders" given FSH early in follicular stimulation.

Summary

Data from 310 patients undergoing follicular stimulation regimes for IVF was evaluated according to 5 stimulation regimes. Three regimes utilised pituitary desensitisation with buserelin, follicular stimulation was induced with either 4 or 6 ampoules of Metrodin and continued with Pergonal in 2 groups, or initiated and continued with Pergonal only. In another group, follicular stimulation occurred using Clomid and Pergonal only, and in the 5th group Metrodin (2 ampoules) and Pergonal only. The outcome of treatment, in terms of pregnancies and live births, was not significantly different between the groups when patient age and the numbers of conceptuses transferred were normalised. The addition of Metrodin in conjunction with buserelin increased the length of the follicular phase, the plasma E_2 and the number of fertilized oocytes. Six ampoules of Metrodin compared to 4 ampoules increased the amount of Pergonal required but the Metrodin "boost" appeared to decrease the amount of Pergonal required for stimulation when compared with Pergonal only. Four ampoules of Metrodin - 2 ampoules on days 1 and 2 of the cycle - proved sufficient. There is no evidence that the addition of Metrodin to follicular stimulation regimes improved overall results and the value of a Metrodin boost remains questionable. However, there was some evidence to suggest that Metrodin may reduce the numbers of cancelled cycles during the follicular phase.

Acknowledgments

We are grateful to our colleagues at the Park Hospital in Nottingham and Rapru, Clinica Nomentana, Rome for their invaluable association with these studies.

Correspondence

To Dr Fishel at the Park Hospital, Nottingham.

References

Bernadus RE, Jones GS, Acosta AA, Garcia JE, Uliu H-C, Jones DL, Rosenwaks Z (1985). The significance of the ratio in follicle stimulating hormone and luteinising hormone in induction of multiple follicular growth. Fertil Steril 43, 373.

Bundren JC, De Cherney AH, Gibbons WE, Marrs RP, Marut EL, Quigley MM, Wentz AC (1990). The use of human follicle-stimulating hormone for ovarian stimulation in in vitro fertilisation. Unpublished data reflecting the results from a multi-centre study; for information contact Serono.

Fishel SB, Edwards RG, Purdy JM, Steptoe PC, Webster J, Walters E, Cohen J, Fehilly C, Hewitt J, Rowland G (1985). Implantation, abortion and birth after in vitro fertilisation using the natural menstrual cycle of follicular stimulation with clomiphene citrate and human menopausal gonadotrophin. J In Vitro Fert. Embryo Transfer 2, 123.

Fishel SB, Jackson P (1989). Follicular stimulation for high tech pregnancies. Are we playing it safe? Br Med J 299, 309.

Jones GS, Acosta AA, Garcia JE, Bernadus RE, Rosenwaks Z (1985). The effect of follicle-stimulating hormone without additional luteinising hormone on follicular stimulation and oocyte development in normal ovulatory women. Fertil. Steril. 43, 696.

Karande VC, Jones GS, Veeck LL, Muasher SJ (1990). High-dose follicle-stimulating hormone stimulation at the onset of the menstrual cycle does not improve the in-vitro fertilisation outcome in low-responder patients. Fertil Steril. 53, 486.

Messinis IE, Templeton AA (1990). The importance of follicle-stimulating hormone increase for folliculogensis. Hum. Reprod. 5, 153.

Navot D & Rosenwaks Z (1988). The use of follicle-stimulating hormone for controlled ovarian hyperstimulation in in vitro fertilisation. J In Vitro Fert. Embryo Transfer 5, 3.

Neveu S, Hedon B, Bringer J, Chinchole J-M, Arnal F, Humeau C, Cristol P, Viala J-L (1987). Of ovarian stimulation by a combination of gonadotrophin-releasing hormone agonist and gonadotrophins for in vitro fertilisation. Fertil Steril 47, 639.

Polan ML, Daniele A, Russell JB, De Cherney AH (1986). Ovulation induction with human menopausal gonadotrophin compared to human urinary follicle-stimulating hormone results in a significant shift in follicular fluid androgen levels without discernible differences in granulosa-luteal cell function. Clin. Endocrinol. Metab. 63, 1284.

GnRH ANALOGUES, PAST PRESENT AND FUTURE USES IN SUPEROVULATION REGIMENS

Introduction

In 1971, the groups of Schally and Guilleman made a major advance in reproductive endocrinology by isolating and determining the structure of gonadotrophin releasing hormone (GnRH). GnRH was found to be a small peptide, just 10 amino acids long. Its duration of biological activity was short, less than 10 minutes. Consequently work was undertaken to synthesise GnRH analogues with a prolonged half-life, which it was hoped could be used to improve fertility by enhancing gonadotrophin output.

Soon after the sequencing of GnRH, analogues were synthesised by altering the natural sequence with other amino acids or more complex molecules. These analogues worked by being "agonistic" to native GnRH and had biological potencies of over 100 times that of the native molecule. Over the last five years some of these agonists have been in routine clinical use for the treatment of hormone-dependent gonadal tumours. However, in the UK, they have also been extensively used in what is still an unlicensed indication, combined with gonadotrophins for inducing multiple follicular development in assisted conception programmes. Their use in this indication will be one of the subjects of the following review.

In comparison, the development of GnRH analogue antagonists for clinical use has been a long and complicated process. The search for an effective antagonist with a very high receptor affinity and an exceptionally long duration of action has resulted in the synthesis of numerous "families" of antagonists. Up to 7 of the 10 natural amino acids have had to be substituted with novel amino acids or D-amino acid residues (Karten and Rivier, 1986) in order to achieve adequate activity.

A further drawback associated with antagonist administration, has been the unacceptably high incidence of side effects such as histamine release. However, recent work has led to the development of a third generation of antagonists, which are potent and remarkably free of side effects. Initial results with third generation antagonists will be briefly discussed.

GnRH Analogue Agonists

The most potent GnRH analogue agonists were those with substitutions at position 6 and 10 of the natural peptide. Table 1 lists a number of commercially available GnRH analogue agonists showing their structure and potency.

Mechanisms of Action

These potentiating substitutions cause an enhanced affinity for the GnRH receptor, thus facilitating the biological activity of the hormone receptor complex. Secondly, the substitutions help protect the analogue from

Table I. Structure and relative potencies of commercially available agonists*

Compound		Structure									Relative Potency
	1	2	3	4	5	6	7	8	9	10	
GnRH	PGlu	His	Trp	Ser	Tyr	Gly	Leu	Arg	Pro	Gly-NH2	1
Buserelin						D-Ser (TBU)				Ethylamide	100
Naferelin						D-(2-Nal)					100
Leuprolide						D-Leu				Ethylamide	50
Goserelin						D-Ser (TBU)				Az-Gly-NH2	50
Decapeptyle						D-Trp					100

* Adapted from Schally and Comaru-Schally (1987).

enzyme degradation thus imparting it with a longer half-life of about 80 minutes (Sandow et al, 1987). An acute injection of one of these superagonists initiates a marked and prolonged release of both luteinising hormone (LH) and follicle stimulating hormone (FSH).

Under normal conditions, the pulsatile discharge of hypothalmic GnRH is essential to stimulate the release of gonadotrophins from the pituitary gonadotrope cells. In the case of continuous GnRH infusion, or chronic administration of GnRH analogue agonists, the pituitary quickly becomes insensitive to further stimulation. This is caused by a loss of occupied GnRH receptors (down-regulation) on the cell surface and an uncoupling

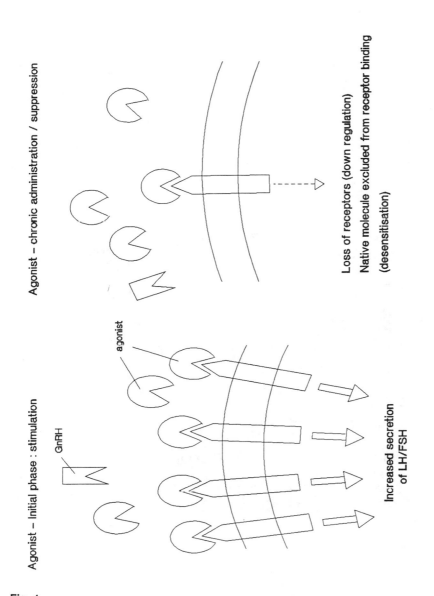

Fig. 1.
Diagrammatic representation of an agonist's interaction with GnRH receptors on the surface of the pituitary gonadotropes.

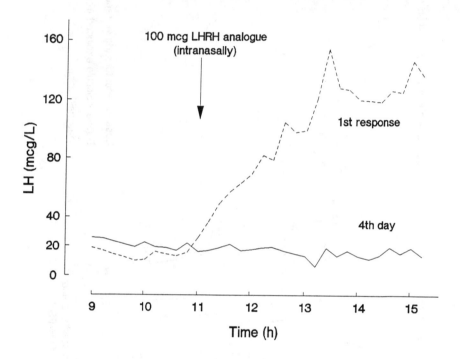

Fig. 2.
Pattern of LH release after the initial administration of the agonist and after four days of treatment (after Shaw et al, 1987).

of the receptors from the secretory signal (desensitisation). These events are represented diagramatically in Fig.1.

These data suggest that gonadotrophin secretion is a function of how the pituitary GnRH receptors "see" and interact with the GnRH molecule. Fig. 2 shows the acute release of gonadotrophins after the initial intranasal administration of 100 mcg agonist and the response to the same dosage on the fourth day of continued four-hourly treatment, (Shaw et al, 1987). It can be seen that the initial flare-up is followed by decreased responsiveness and finally, inhibition of gonadotrophin secretion.

Thus, a pharmacological and reversible hypophysectomy (or transient medical castration) can be achieved without affecting the release of other pituitary hormones. Spontaneous pituitary and gonadal activity quickly returns once GnRH analogue agonist administration is discontinued (Fraser et al, 1987).

Routes of Administration

GnRH analogue agonists can be administered via three routes, subcutaneous, intranasal or as a depot injection. Each route has its limitations, with regard to use in superovulation regimens. For instance, daily subcutaneous injections may limit clinical acceptability and reduce patient compliance.

Intranasal insufflation also has its problems. Absorption is reduced, (300 mcg intranasally is equivalent in action to 10 mcg subcutaneously; Sandow et al, 1987) with the dose being required several times a day in order to achieve the desired biological effect. Compliance has also been recognised as a problem (Rajfer et al, 1986) as well as drug absorption being unacceptably variable (Furr, 1987).

Depot formulations probably offer a more convenient method of delivering analogue agonist over a protracted period of time. These preparations consist of the agonist microencapsulated in a biodegradable material such as poly (DL-lactide-CO-glycolide). Current formulations release drug over about 30 days. However this length of use is inappropriate for superovulation regimens. For instance, if the luteal phase of the cycle falls in the period of suppression and the patient becomes pregnant, prolonged luteal support will be required.

Although depot formulations were developed to increase clinical and patient compliance, it has been found that they offer improved efficacy. Within 6-8h blood concentrations of the agonist have reached steady state conditions (Sandow, 1987). Further, the depots cause a higher degree of pituitary desensitisation (Furr, 1987). In relation to superovulation therefore, the ideal mode of administration, from a patient viewpoint, is intranasal. Clinically, subcutaneous injections are more economical and more readily achieve a state of relative ovarian quiescence. A single dose of 500 mcg daily is sufficient to induce consistent pituitary receptor downregulation throughout the day (Sandow and Donnez, 1989). Depot formulations on the other hand induce a deep state of pituitary desensitisation, which is achieved faster than other regimens employing frequent bolus dosing (Lemay et al, 1986; Matta et al, 1988). This deeper state of pituitary quiescence may have important implications for the choice of gonadotrophin used in inducing follicular development.

Extra-Pituitary Effects

Reproductive toxicology and teratogenecity studies, carried out on the GnRH agonist buserelin, have revealed no teratogenic effects in a number of mammalian species (Akaike et al, 1987 a,b). Inadvertent use during pregnancy has been reported to cause minimal risk for fetal development. The available worldwide results to date, of the use of agonists in assisted conception procedures, have not reported any association with congenital malformations, (various authors, 1989). However, bioactive GnRH agonist has been found to concentrate in human follicular fluid (Loumaye et al, 1989). Further, the presence of low affinity GnRH receptors in the human ovary, have been reported (Bramley et al, 1985).

The significance of these findings, in relation to the use of agonists for superovulation are as yet unknown, but Loumaye et al (1989) suggested that administration should be stopped before oocytes are collected.

Recent research has suggested a possible beneficial effect of agonist on the endometrium. Steer and colleagues (1989) reported a significantly higher pregnancy rate in women undergoing a frozen embryo replacement in an agonist/HRT cycle. They hypothesised that the agonist may slow down the rate of endometrial development. This retardation may increase the period of receptivity and hence, improve the chances of pregnancy. Further work is in progress to try and demonstrate the presence of GnRH receptors in the endometrium.

Rationale for the use of GnRH Analogue Agonists in Superovulation Regimens

The impetus for the use of GnRH agonists in the treatment of infertile women stemmed from the pioneering work of Fleming et al (1982). They first reported the use of agonists, in combination with gonadotrophins, for the treatment of patients with abnormal hormone profiles. Subsequent work was carried out in women with different aetiologies of infertility. Under these circumstances, ovulation induction was carried out without interference from endogenous LH (Fleming et al, 1985; Fleming and Coutts, 1986), thereby eliminating premature (pre-hCG) luteinisation (Fleming et al, 1985) and improving the patients' chance of achieving a pregnancy.

Following on from these observations, there have been a plethora of reports, from IVF and ovulation induction studies, suggesting that the viability of embryos derived from oocytes exposed to inappropriate LH levels may be adversely affected (IVF: Stanger and Yovich, 1985; Howles et al, 1986; Punnonen et al, 1988: Ovulation induction: Abdulwahid et al, 1985; Homburg et al, 1988). If these compromised embryos implant, they are more likely to result in an early miscarriage (Homburg et al, 1988; Regan et al, 1989; Watson et al, 1989; Johnson and Pearce, 1990). Thus, abnormal follicular endocrinology may be a casual factor, not only for implantation failure, but also in early pregnancy loss.

A further problem encountered in stimulated cycles is the occurence of the LH surge. Up to 20% of the patients undergo an endogenous LH surge (Macnamee et al, 1988). The use of gonadotrophins alone or in combination with clomiphene citrate results in an attenuation of the LH surge (Messinis et al, 1985) making it difficult to detect. Intensive endocrine monitoring is required, so that if a surge does occur it is detected and the appropriate action taken. Under some circumstances, the strength of the surge may only be sufficient to induce oocyte maturation but not follicular rupture. Thus, luteinised unruptured follicle syndrome may be a common problem in stimulated cycles, (Howles and Macnamee, 1989). By employing the agonist, problems of both raised tonic LH and the occurence of the LH surge, can be adequately controlled. Furthermore, the clinician can plan oocyte retrievals to occur during the working day and not at weekends (Zorn et al, 1987; Rutherford et al, 1988). It is not surprising therefore, that use of agonists in superovulation regimens, has gained such popularity. They have contributed significantly to the recent increase in success rates of assisted conception treatment cycles.

Superovulation Regimens Employing the Agonist

The earliest paper on the use of agonists in combination with gonadotrophins for IVF, reported a benefit in women who proved resistant to other forms of stimulation (Porter et al, 1984). This was followed by a report, on the establishment of a twin IVF pregnancy, after agonist treatment combined with pure FSH (Shaw et al, 1985). Since these early reports, there has been a widespread acceptance of the agonist as a prerequisite to superovulation, not only for the treatment of known poor responders (eg Schmitz et al, 1987; Rutherford et al 1988; MacLachlen et al 1989) but also for patients with normal endocrine function (eg Macnamee et al, 1989).

To date, there are three regimens in clinical practice. These involve either an extended period of ovarian suppression prior to gonadotrophin treatment (long protocol); a two to three day delay between first administration of the agonist and gonadotrophins (short protocol), or just a brief three day exposure of the patient to the agonist (ultra-short) followed by gonadotrophins. These regimens are summarised in Table II.

Table II. Summary of superovulation protocols utilising agonists.

Protocol	Drug	Administration
Long protocol	Agonist	Day 1 or 21 of menstrual cycle. Continue until hCG
	Gonadotrophins	Depends upon criteria used to determine pituitary/ovarian inactivity. A delay of 14 days is not un-common
Short protocol	Agonist	Day 1-3 of menstrual cycle. Continue until hCG
	Gonadotrophins	1 or 2 days after start of agonist
Ultrashort protocol	Agonist	Day 1 or 2 of menstrual cycle for 3 days (500 mcg/day sc)
	Gonadotrophins	Day 2 of agonist

The long and short protocol are similar in that agonist is administered up until hCG is given to induce final follicular maturation. The does of agonist administered varies according to the route of administration. Common doses employed, via intranasal insufflation, range from 100 mcg to 300 mcg given five times per day, (every four hours excluding the 3.00 am dose; Shaw et al, 1985; Rutherford et al, 1988). Daily subcutaneous doses commonly used range from a 200 mcg bolus (Tan et al, personal communication), to 300 mcg twice daily (Neveu et al, 1987; Frydman et al, 1988). However in the ultrashort protocol, 500 mcg/day are given subcutaneously for only three days (Howles et al, 1987; Sharma et al, 1988) starting on day 1 or 2 of the treatment cycle.

Long Protocol

The long protocol can either be started in the late luteal phase of the previous cycle (day 21 or day 22, Shaw et al, 1985), or on day 1 or 2 of the cycle (Neveu et al, 1987). Administration of agonist in the late luteal phase, has a transient luteotrophic effect (Fleming and Coutts, 1982) and results in a significantly lower flare-up and a more rapid decrease in circulating gonadotrophins (MacLachlan et al, 1989). However, there is no evidence to suggest that the outcome of the treatment cycle is affected by starting the agonist in the luteal or early follicular phase.

In the vast majority of reported cases, whether the patients are poor responders, PCOD's or endocrinologically normal, gonadotrophins are administered from about the second week of agonist treatment. The criteria used for initiation of gonadotrophins vary, from purely ultrasonic (eg regression of all ovarian follicles to less than 5mm diameter and or no endometrial echo), to solely biochemical and in some cases a combination of the two. Some examples are shown in Table III. It is notable that some of these criteria are extremely strict. It is questionable therefore, whether such stringent criteria are really necessary. As illustrated in Fig. 2, gonadotrophin secretion returns to baseline values within four days of initiating agonist treatment. As the purpose of pituitary desensitisation is solely to keep LH within the normal follicular range, and as long as progesterone is not elevated (ie no ovarian cystic structures are present), there seems little need to wait for extended periods to initiate gonadotrophin therapy.

Table III. Start criteria for gonadotrophins in long agonist protocols.

Start day of agonist	Start day of monitoring	Criteria	Reference
2	11	Plasma E2 and ultrasound	Frydman et al, 1987
1 or 2	14	Urinary E and ultrasound	Neveu et al, 1988
1	15	Ultrasound	Jacobs et al, 1987
Varied		E2 < 180pmol/l for 3 days	MacLachlan et al, 1989
2	14	E2 < 100pmol/l, LH < 3U/L and ultrasound	Rutherford et al, 1988

However, it has been reported that menses can occur about 12 days (range 9-16) after the beginning of agonist treatment in the early follicular phase (MacLachlan et al, 1989). In these cases it would obviously be unwise to initiate gonadotrophin stimulation until menstruation had occurred. However this observation has not been documented consistently by other workers using the follicular phase long protocol (eg Rutherford et al, 1988).

Thus it would seem that starting agonist in the luteal phase may be a better choice. The onset of menses could be used as a reliable indicator of pituitary/ovarian quiescence thus signallying the start of gonadotrophin therapy. However the period of hypogonadotrophic hypogonadism may be extended to allow for cycle programming (Rutherford et al, 1988).

Short Protocols

The short or "flare-up" and ultra short protocols are started on day 1 to 3 of the cycle (Barriere et al, 1987; Howles et al, 1987 and Frydman et al, 1988). These protocols utilise the flare-up effect to initiate follicular recruitment, which can reduce the cost of treatment. There has been a great deal of debate on the relative merits of the long versus short protocols. Loumaye et al (1989), compared the hormonal changes and fertilization rates in nine patients on a short and long protocol. Progesterone concentrations in the short protocol were elevated above normal, for 4 days after the start of agonist administrations. They concluded that short protocols were associated with reduced fertilization rates and embryo quality. This is in contrast for example to another study which utilised an ultra-short protocol (Macnamee et al, 1989).

It has been recommended that ultrasound scanning of the ovary is carried out in order to identify the presence of any cystic structures prior to agonist administration in short protocols (Howles et al, 1987). This precautionary step was advocated, in view of evidence to suggest that the flare-up phenomenon may cause rescue of the old corpus luteum resulting in inappropriate progesterone secretion during follicular stimulation (Fleming et al, 1987).

Further data from this group suggests that, in short protocols started on day 3, the flare-up effect can cause luteinisation of developing antral follicles (Fleming et al, personal communication).

It seems appropriate therefore that some form of monitoring whether it be ultrasound visualisation of the ovaries and/or progesterone determinations should be carried out around the onset of agonist administration in short or ultra-short protocols. If cystic structures are visualised or progesterone is elevated, then gonadotrophin administration should be delayed until ovarian inactivity returns.

This problem can however be alleviated by pre-administration of norethisterone, which causes a state of ovarian quiescence. Such a combination has been suggested by Zorn and colleagues (1987) to allow for the programming of IVF and GIFT treatment cycles. Here, norethisterone was given 10 mg daily from day 2 of a spontaneous cycle for 7 to 25 days, always ending on a Monday. On the subsequent Friday (first day of stimulation), a single dose of a depot agonist as well as HMG were administered. Out of 119 oocyte recoveries carried out, 116 were performed on Wednesday, three on Saturday and none on Sunday.

A second problem associated with the use of short protocols in certain patient groups, is that gonadotrophin secretion may not return to baseline values during stimulation. Luteinising hormone may still be inappropriately high, during the LH sensitive stages of late follicular phase. For instance, PCO patients take on average seven days longer than control patients to return within the normal LH range after the start of buserelin therapy (Fleming et al, 1987).

In summary, in spite of these caveats short protocols have been successfully employed for the treatment of poor responders and normal patients (Howles et al, 1987; Macnamee et al, 1989). However more intensive monitoring of the cycle is required and patient selection is more critical for a successful outcome, than in long protocols.

Factors Affecting the Success of Agonist Protocols

Criteria for hCG administration

A recent study has suggested that the traditional criteria for giving hCG (based on clomiphene citrate and gonadotrophin treatment cycles) should be reassessed when agonists are employed (Conaghan et al, 1989). Conaghan et al (1989) reported significantly higher pregnancy rates if the administration of hCG was delayed by at least 24 hours after the normal criteria was met (3 largest follicles are over 17mm in diameter with appropriate oestradiol values for the number of follicles visualised).

In clomiphene/gonadotrophin cycles, hCG may have been timed early in order to avoid the incidence of an endogenous LH surge. Thus, by delaying hCG administration in agonist cycles, follicles are growing on to the size they would normally reach in spontaneous cycles.

Type and dose of gonadotrophin used for superovulation

One of the first reports of a successful IVF pregnancy after agonist treatment was obtained with pure FSH (METRODIN) (Shaw et al, 1985). In a small number of comparative studies, there was no difference between the pregnancy rates obtained between patients who received pure FSH or HMG (Bentick et al, 1988; Frydman et al, 1987). Neveu et al (1988) reported that although the pregnancy rate was high (60%), oestrogen levels were significantly lower in patients given agonist combined with FSH compared to those receiving FSH alone.

This observation is in accord with the two cell, two gonadotrophin theory of steroidogenesis. Both LH and FSH are required for normal oestrogen secretion. The lowered oestrogen output suggests that the amount of LH available for thecal cell androgen production was reduced, however oocyte quality was not compromised.

It can be concluded that, although tonic LH secretion is reduced by the use of subcutaneous or nasal spray agonist administration, there is sufficient bioactive LH still present for normal follicular development. However, this may not be the case if a depot agonist is utilised. As mentioned earlier, the level of pituitary desensitisation after depot administration is greater resulting in a deeper suppression of LH output. Under these conditions it is possible that some exogenous LH (in the form of HMG) will be required. However this is currently only speculation. Clinical studies are required to identify how much LH is needed during follicular development.

A major effect of employing agonists in superovulation regimens is the increase in cost per treatment cycle. Long protocols can increase gonadotrophin consumption by at least 70% (from approximately 14 ampoules in CC/HMG cycles to 24 or more ampoules/cycle). As agonists reduce gonadotrophin secretion it will be necessary to raise endogenous levels of FSH again, to the minimum threshold value required to initiate follicular recruitment.

However, the length of stimulation does not seem to be significantly increased compared to clomiphene/gonadotrophin cycles (eg approximately 11 days for long protocol, Bentick et al, 1987).

In spite of this increase in drug expenditure, the overall cost-effectiveness of agonist regimens is greatly improved. Fewer cycles are cancelled (Rutherford et al, 1988), and oocyte recoveries can be programmed to occur within working hours and not at weekends (Zorn et al, 1987; Rutherford et al, 1988). Most importantly the pregnancy rates per treatment cycle are significantly improved over CC/HMG cycles. However, one drawback is the possibility of a higher multiple pregnancy rate after agonist treatment (Rutherford et al, 1988).

Luteal phase support

Smitz et al (1987) suggested that the corpora lutea generated after agonist/gonadotrophin may be functionally defective. For this reason, they advocated support of the early luteal phase with hCG injections. Recently, Smith et al (1989) in a randomised trial showed that support of the luteal phase with hCG was associated with a significantly higher implantation rate. However great care should be taken to avoid initiating ovarian hyperstimulation syndrome through luteal hCG injections.

Ovarian hyperstimulation syndrome

Ovarian hyperstimulation syndrome (OHSS) is one of the most serious of the complications affecting superovulation. In its most severe form, hospitalisation is required and evidence is now accumulating that the incidence of OHSS may actually be increased after agonist administration (Golan et al, 1988; Barlow, 1988). Whether the increased incidence of OHSS is due to excessive stimulation is not known. However as most cases of OHSS are associated with pregnancy and as the pregnancy rate is increased by the use of agonists, OHSS may be an unavoidable consequence of agonist therapy.

It has been suggested that in cases where OHSS is anticipated (eg rapidly rising oestradiol levels during the follicular phase), gonadotrophins should be stopped, but agonist continued until the follicles have completely regressed (Fleming, personal communication).

GnRH Analogue Antagonists

Mechanisms of Action

In contrast to the agonists, GnRH antagonists act by competing with GnRH for the receptor binding site, without causing an activation of the bound receptor and release of gonadotrophins.

This results in an immediate inhibition of gonadotrophin secretion. Thus, there would be advantages in certain clinical situations of employing an antagonist rather than an agonist.

Side Effects

As initmated in the Introduction, the development of potent GnRH antagonists has been slow and problematical. Part of the problem relates to the more complex and extensive modifications of the natural molecule required to achieve antagonistic function. High doses have been required to compete successfully with endogenous GnRH. This made some of the early antagonists only suitable for indications in which short term, rapid effects are required. Further, the "first generation" antagonists induced histamine release in vitro (Hock et al, 1985) and oedema and inflamation at the injection site (Schmidt et al, 1984) in animals.

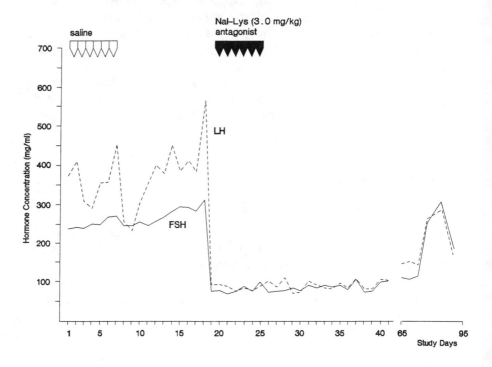

Fig. 3.
Pattern of gonadotrophin secretion in an ovariectomised monkey administered
Antide (3 mg/kg) and control saline injections as indicated by key.

Clinical Effects of the Antagonists

Because of these side-effects, few clinical trials have been carried out in humans. However using a weak antagonist, it was observed that administration in women for 3 days, resulted in an increase in the length of the follicular phase (Mais et al, 1986).

Further studies in women using a second generation antagonist (Nal-Glu) resulted in a prolongation of the follicular phase by 10 days (Bouchard et al, 1989). This was due to a demise in the dominant follicle and the subsequent selection and growth of a new dominant follicle. However, in an earlier study using this antagonist, local allergic responses in some human subjects was a concern (Pavlou et al, 1987).

The demonstration in a third generation antagonist of negligible histamine release properties coupled with a high potency, has at last heralded the start of a major research programme which it is hoped will at last lead to an antagonist in routine clinical use.

This antagonist, called Antide (Nal-Lys) has been found to exhibit some interesting properties. Studies in primates have shown that sc or iv administration of Antide causes an unexpectedly prolonged inhibition of gonadotrophin secretion (Leal et al, 1988). Further it was found that, even after an iv injection of Antide (3 mg/kg) levels remained in the peripheral circulation for up to 40 days (Fig. 3, Danforth et al, 1989). These data suggest that the highly hydrophobic Antide is protected from enzymatic degradation and elimination by binding to serum proteins (Danforth et al, in press). Other antagonists have also been reported to bind to such proteins (Davis et al, 1987).

Table IV. Time to reach pretreatment LH/FSH concentration in long-term ovariectomised monkeys administered antagonists.

Treatment Group	Monkey	Days to reach pretreatment values	
		LH	FSH
Nal-Glu (2nd gen) 1.0 mg/kg/day	27	21	17
	33	22	21
*Nal-Lys 0.3 mg/kg/day	28	23	22
	29	45	10
*Nal-Lys 1.0 mg/kg/day	1	62	62
	31	45	45
*Nal-Lys 3.0 mg/kg.day	32	100	100
	27	62	62

  * Antide, 3rd generation GnRH antagonist

The long duration of action by Antide is also highly dose dependent (Table IV). A dose of 0.3 mg/kg was found to be equivalent to approximately 1.0 mg/kg of the second generation antagonist, Nal-Glu.

Another interesting feature is the reversal of gonadotrophin suppression by iv injections of exogenous GnRH (Hodgen et al, in press). This reversal occurred at the highest dose of Antide used. These data suggest that Antide promises to be a highly potent dose dependent antagonist (with negligible side effects) which could be utilised for a wide number of clinical applications.

Summary

The widespread adoption of GnRH analogue agonists in superovulation regimens has been one of the most significant advances in assisted conception over the last three years. Although analogue use increases the cost per treatment cycle, the number of cancelled cycles are reduced. Further oocyte collections can be planned according to workload and carried out during working hours. Also, monitoring for an LH surge is not required. Further and most importantly, pregnancy rates are increased.

The use of antagonists in clinical practice is eagerly awaited, however it is too early to assign a role for them in assisted conception cycles. Major clinical trials are required to fully elucidate their mechanisms of action.

References

Abdulwahid NA, Adams J, Van de Spuy ZM and Jacobs HS (1985). Gonadotrophin control of follicular development. Clin. Endocrinol., 23, 613-626.

Akaike M, Takayama K, Ohno H, et al (1987a). Teratogenicity study of subcutaneously administered buserelin acetate in mice. Pharmacometrics, 33, 631-640.

Akaike M, Takayama K, Ohno H, et al (1987b). Teratogenicity study of subcutaneously administered buserelin acetate in rabbits. Pharmacometrics, 33, 641-646.

Barlow D (1988). Letter to the editor - In Vitro Fertilisation. Brit. Med. J., 297, 201.

Barriere P, Lopes P, Boiffard JP, et al (1987). Use of GnRH analogues in ovulation induction for in vitro fertilisation: benefit of a short administration regimen. J. In Vitro. Fert. Embryo Transfer, 4, 64-65.

Barron JL, Millar R and Searle D (1982). Metabolic clearance and plasma half-disappearance time of D-Trp[6] and exogenous luteinising hormone releasing hormone. J. Clin. Endocrinol. Metab., 54, 1169-1173.

Bentick B, Shaw RW, Iffland CA, et al (1988). A randomized comparative study of purified follicle stimulating hormone and human menopausal gonadotrophin after pituitary desensitization with Buserelin for superovulation and in vitro fertilisation. Fertil. Steril., 50, 79-84.

Bouchard P, Wolf JP and Hajari S (1988). Inhibition of ovulation: comparison between the mechanism of action of steriods and GnRH analogues. Hum. Reprod. 3, 503-506.

Bramley TA, Menzies GS and Baird DT (1985). Specific binding of gonadotrophin-releasing hormone and an agonist to human corpus luteum homogenates: characterization, properties, and luteal phase levels. J. Clin. Endocrinol. Metab., 61, 834-841.

Conaghan J, Dimitry ES, Mills M, et al (1989). Delayed human chorionic gonadotrophin administration for in-vitro fertilisation. Lancet, i, 1323-1324.

Danforth DR, Gordon K, Leal JA, et al (1990). Extended presence of Antide (Nal-Lys GnRH antagonist) in circulation: prolonged duration of gonadotrophin inhibition may derive from Antide binding to serum proteins. J. Clin. Endocrinol. Metab. (in press).

Danforth D, Williams R, Gordon K and Hodgen G (1989). Development of an in vitro bioassay for GnRH antagonists: measurement of circulating Nal-Lys GnRH antagonist levels to examine the mechanism of its long action. 22nd annual meeting of the Society for the Study of Reproduction, Abstr. 364.

Fleming R, Adam AH, Barlow DH, et al (1982). A new systematic treatment for infertile women with abnormal hormone profiles. Brit. J. Obstet, Gynaecol., 89, 80-83.

Fleming R and Coutts JRT (1986). Induction of multiple follicular growth in normally menstruating women with endogenous gonadotrophin suppression. Fertil. Steril., 45, 226-230.

Fleming R, Haxton MJ, Hamilton MPR, et al (1985). Successful treatment of infertile women with oligomenorrhoea using a combination of an LHRH agonist and exogenous gonadotrophins. Brit. J. Obstet. Gynaecol., 92, 369-373.

Fraser HM, Yorkston CE, Sandow J, et al (1987). The biological evaluation of LHRH agonists (buserelin) implants in the female stumptailed macaque. Brit. J. Clin. Pract., 41, (Suppl. 48), 14-21.

Frydman R, Belaisch-Allart J, Parneix, I, et al (1988). Comparison between flare up and down regulation effects of luteinizing hormone-releasing hormone agonists in an in vitro fertilisation program. Fertil. Steril., 50, 471-475.

Furr BJA (1987). Pharmacological studies with Zoladex, a novel luteinizing hormone-releasing hormone analogue. In: Zoladex - a new treatment for prostatic cancer, GD Chisholm (ed), P. 1-15, RSM Services Ltd., London.

Golan A, Ron-El R, Herman A, et al (1988). Ovarian hyperstimulation syndrome following D-Trp-6 luteinizing hormone-releasing hormone microcapsules and menotropin for in vitro fertilization. Fertil. Steril., 50, 912-916.

Hook WA, Karten M and Siraganian RP (1985). Histamine released by structural analogs of LHRH. Fed. Proc., 44, (No. 5336).

Homburg R, Armar NA, Eshel A, et al (1988). Influence of serum luteinising hormone concentrations on ovulation, conception and early pregnancy loss in polycystic ovary syndrome. Brit. Med. J., 297, 1024-1026.

Howles CM and Macnamee MC (1990). The endocrinology of stimulated cycles: influence on outcome. 5th World Congress on IVF and Alternate Assisted Reproduction, Academic Press (in press).

Howles CM, Macnamee MC, Edwards RG et al (1986). Effect of high tonic levels of luteinising hormone on outcome of in-vitro fertilisation. Lancet, ii, 521-522.

Howles CM, Macnamee MC and Edwards RG (1987). Short term use of LHRH agonist to treat poor responders entering an in-vitro fertilization (IVF) programme. Hum. Reprod., 2, 655-656.

Jacobs HS, Porter RN, Eshel A, et al (1987). Profertility uses of LHRH agonist analogues. In: LHRH and its analogues: contraception and therapeutic application II, BH Vickery, JJ Nector (eds), MTP Press, Lancaster, 303-319.

Johnson P and Pearce JM (1990). Recurrent spontaneous abortion and polycycstic ovarian disease: comparison of two regimens to induce ovulation. Brit. Med. J., 300, 154-156.

Karten MJ and Rivier JE (1986). Gonadotrophin-releasing hormone analog design. Structure-function studies toward the development of agonists and antagonists. Rationale and persepctives. Endocrinol. Rev., 7, 44-52.

Leal JA, Gordon K, Williams RF, et al (1990). Probing studies on multiple dose effects of Antide (Nal-Lys) GnRH antagonist in ovariectomized monkeys. Contraception (in press).

Lemay A, Maheux R, Clement J and Faure N (1986). Efficacy of different modalities of LHRH agonist (buserelin) administation on the inhibition of the pituitary-ovarian axis for the treatment of endometriosis. In: Gonado-trophin down-regulation in clinical practice, R Rolland, DR Chadha and WN Willemsen (eds), Alan R Liss, New York, p.157.

Loumaye E, Coen G, Pampfer S, et al (1989). Use of a gonadotrophin-re-leasing hormone agonist during ovarian stimulation leads to significant concentrations of peptide in follicular fluids. Fertil. Steril., 52, 256-263.

Loumaye E, Vankrieken L, Depreester S, et al (1989). Hormonal changes induced by short-term administration of a gonadotrophin-releasing hor-mone agonist during ovarian hyperstimulation for in vitro fertilisation and their consequences for embryo development. Fertil. Steril., 51, 105-111.

MacLachlan V, Besanko M, O'Shea F, et al (1989). A controlled study of luteinizing hormone-releasing hormone agonist (buserelin) for the induc-tion of folliculogenesis before in vitro fertilization. N. Engl. J. Med., 320, 1233-1237.

Macnamee MC, Howles CM and Edwards RG (1987). The effects of ovarian stimulation on endogenous endocrine rhythms. In: The control of follicle development, ovulation and luteal function: Lessons from IVF, F Naftolin and AH De Cherney (eds), Serono Symposia 35, Raven Press, New York, p.121.

Macnamee MC, Howles CM, Edwards RG, et al (1989). Short-term luteinizing hormone relasing hormone agonist treatment: prospective trial of a novel ovarian stimulation regimen for in vitro fertilisation. Fertil. Steril., 52, 264-269.

Mais V, Kazer RR, Cetel NS, et al (1986). The dependency of folliculogen-esis and corpus luteum function on pulsatile gonadotrophin secretion in cycling women using a GnRH antagonist as a probe. J. Clin. Endocrinol. Metab., 62, 1250-1255.

Matta WHM, Shaw RW and Burford GD (1988). Endocrinologic and clinical evaluation following a single administration of a gonadotrophin-releasing hormone agonist (Zoladex), in a depot formulation, to premenopausal women. Fertil. Steril., 49, 163-165.

Messinis IE, Templeton AA and Baird DT (1985). Endogenous luteinizing hormone surge during superovulation induction with sequential use of clomiphene citrate and pulsatile human menopausal gonadotrophin. J. Clin. Endocrinol. Metab., 61, 1076-1081.

Neveu S, Hedon B, Bringer J, et al (1987). Ovarian stimulation by a combination of a gonadotrophin-releasing hormone agonist and gonado-trophins for in vitro fertilisation. Fertil. Steril., 47, 639-643.

Pavlou SN, Wakefield GB, Island DP, et al (1987). Suppression of pituitary-gonadal function by a potent new luteinizing hormone-releasing hormone antagonist in normal men. J. Clin. Endocrinol. Metab., 64, 931-936.

Porter RN, Smith W, Craft IL, et al (1984). Induction of ovulation for in-vitro fertilisation using buserelin and gonadotrophins. Lancet, ii, 1284-1285.

Punnonen R, Ashorn R, Vilja P, et al (1988). Spontaneous luteinizing hormone surge and cleavage of in-vitro fertilized embryos. Fertil. Steril., 49, 479-482.

Rajfer J, Handelsman FJ, Crum A, et al (1986). Comparison of the efficacy of subcutaneous and nasal spray buserelin treatment in suppression of testicular steriodogenesis in men with prostate cancer. Fertil. Steril., 46, 104-110.

Regan L, Owen EJ and Jacobs HS (1989). Hypersecretion of LH and Spontaneous Miscarriage: A Field Study. J. Endocrinol., Suppl. 123, ab 28.

Rutherford AJ, Subak-Sharpe RJ, Dawson KJ, et al (1988). Improvement of in vitro fertilisation after treatment with buserelin, an agonist of luteinis-ing hormone releasing hormone. Brit. Med. J., 296, 1765-1768.

Rutherford AJ, Subak-Sharpe RJ, Dawson KJ, et al (1988). Programmed IVF treatment using Buserelin/HMG for superovulation. Fourth Meeting of ESHRE, Barcelona, ab 187.

Sandow J (1990). The clinical use of LHRH agonists. P Steptoe Memorial Symposium "Establishment of a human pregnancy", Ares Serono Symposia, Raven Press, New York, (in press).

Sandow J and Donnez J (1989). Clinical pharmacokinetics of LHRH analogues. In: The present place of LHRH in gynaecology. Parthenon Publishing, Lancaster (in press).

Sandow J, Fraser HM, Seidel H et al (1987). Buserelin: Pharmacokinetics, metabolism and mechanisms of action. Brit. J. Clin. Pract., 41, (Suppl. 48) 6-13.

Schally AV and Comaru-Schally AM (1987). Use of luteinizing hormone-releasing hormone analogs in the treatment of hormone dependent tumors. Seminars Reprod. Endocrinol., 5, 389-397.

Schmidt F, Sundaram K, Thau RB, Bardin CW (1984). (Ac-D-Nal (2)[1], 4FD-Phe[2], D-Trp[3], D-Arg[6]) - LHRH, a potent antagonist of LHRH, produces transient edema and behavioural changes in rats. Contraception, 29, 283.

Sharma V, Williams J, Collins W, et al (1987). A comparison of treatments with exogenous FSH to promote folliculogensis in patients with quiescent ovaries due to the continued administration of an LHRH agonist. Hum. Reprod., 2, 553-556.

Sharma V, Williams J, Collins W, et al (1988). The sequential use of a luteinizing hormone-releasing hormone (LH-RH) agonist and human menopausal gonadotrophins to stimulate folliculogenesis in patients with resistant ovaries. J. In Vitro Fertil. Embryo Transfer, 5, 38-42.

Shaw RW, Ndukwe G, Imoedemhe DAG, et al (1985). Twin pregnancy after pituitary desensitisation with LHRH agonist and pure FSH. Lancet, ii, 506.

Shaw RW, Ndukwe G, Imoedemhe DAG, et al (1987). Endocrine changes following pituitary desensitization with LHRH agonist and adminstration of purified FSH to induce follicular maturation. Brit. J. Obstet. Gynaecol., 94, 682-686.

Smith EM, Anthony FW, Gadd SC and Masson GM (1989). Trial of support treatment with human chorionic gonadotrophin in the luteal phase after treatment with buserelin and human menopausal gonadotrophin in women taking part in an in vitro fertilisation programme. Brit. Med. J., 298, 1483-1486.

Smitz J, Devroey P, Braeckmans P, et al (1987). Management of failed cycles in an IVF/GIFT programme with the combination of a GnRH analogue and HMG. Hum. Reprod., 2, 309-314.

Stanger JD and Yovich JL (1985). Reduced in vitro fertilization of human oocytes from patients with raised basal luteinizing hormone levels during the follicular phase. Br. J. Obstet. Gynaecol., 92, 385-393.

Steer C, Mason BA, Sathanadan M, et al (1989). Pituitary-ovarian axis down regulation with LHRH agonist therapy increases frozen embryo pregnancy rates. Symposium on Neuroendocrine Regulation of Reproduction, Serono Symposia, USA, Abstr. 41.

Various authors (1989). Plennary session: World collaborative results and outcome of IVF pregnancies. VI World congress IVF and Alternate Assisted Reproduction, Jerusalem.

Vickery BH and Nector JJ (1987). Luteinizing hormone-releasing hormone analogs: developments and mechanisms of action. Seminars Reprod. Endocrinol., 5, 353-369.

Watson, H, Hamilton-Fairley D, Kiddy D, et al (1989). Abnormalities of follicular phase LH secretion in women with recurrent early miscarriage. J. Endocrinol., Suppl. 123, ab 25.

Zorn JR, Boyer P, Guichard A (1987). Never on a Sunday: programming for IVF-ET and GIFT. Lancet, i, 385-386.

5 *D.H. Barlow, D.Egan, C. Ross*

THE OUTCOME OF IVF PREGNANCY

Introduction

Infertile couples faced with the possibility of using assisted conception can easily be confused by the variety of types of statistic which might be presented to them both by doctors and the lay media. At present they may be asked to consider whether treatments such as IUI, GIFT, ZIFT or IVF might be appropriate for their particular needs. Leaving aside differences in patient selection, sample sizes and methodology which can undermine meaningful comparison between statistics from different units, couples (and professionals) can be misled by the variety of numerators and denominators used. Most workers in IVF would now agree that biochemical pregnancies (resulting in preclinical abortion) should be omitted from statistics and that success should preferably be quoted in terms of treatment cycles commenced where possible. There is a tendency to quote GIFT results in terms of laparoscopies performed which gives GIFT results a favourable gloss compared with those for IVF.

The couple come to IVF in order to have a baby thus, although it is helpful to be able to quote the chance of having a pregnancy which can be confirmed ultrasonically if they start a treatment cycle, this is not entirely answering the questions usually uppermost in their mind. The important questions are "how likely are we to have a baby if we have a treatment attempt?" and "how likely would it be if we persist for several attempts?" Matters such as the stress involved in IVF, the costs of IVF, how they would cope with treatment failure etc cannot be overlooked but if the couple cannot be given appropriate statistics they cannot make the best decision for their situation. Appropriate statistics must allow for the significant losses which occur even after the happy confirmation of the pregnancy at the first scan.

In considering the outcome of IVF pregnancies the results of the IVF Unit at the John Radcliffe Hospital will be included as an example of a large experience of pregnancy outcome principally involving long protocol buserelin controlled cycles (762 cycles) on a uniform treatment protocol. Since this type of protocol is probably the commonest in current British use and since all of the pregnancies described occurred after April 1987 it is a description of what can be achieved today whereas many of the important papers on pregnancy outcome relate to older IVF experience which might not be so representative of current outcomes.

The Oxford data from April 1987 to September 1988 covers 1,011 consecutive treatment cycles. From April 1988 all cycles have involved GnRH analogue control whereas in the first year the standard protocol was Clomiphene/Pergonal with Norethisterone scheduling (249 cycles) and only "problem cases" received the analogue (Barlow et al, 1988).

SPONTANEOUS ABORTION

Spontaneous abortion has been regarded as a problem in IVF treatment as can be seen in the results of the first 100 births from the Clamart Unit in France (Frydman et al, 1986). The spontaneous abortion rate was 22.5% and the ectopic rate 2.5%, both typical of many IVF reports. Yovich and Matson (1988) examined these rates in a range of infertility problems and demonstrated that similar rates of loss occurred with different levels of manipulation of reproduction (Table 1). The spontaneous abortion rate

Table 1 Pregnancy Wastage after Gamete Manipulation (from Yovich & Matson, 1988).

Treatment	n	B.O. %	Misc. %	Ect. %	Del. > 19 %
Unstim.	462	12.1	5.0	5.0	75.3
Stim.	175	15.4	6.9	5.1	69.7
AIH	76	19.7	4.0	5.3	67.1
AID	116	11.2	4.3	0.9	81.9
GIFT	76	7.9	6.6	9.2	67.1
IVF	119	14.3	0.8	7.6	68.1

after IVF was 15.1% which is not likely to be higher than in natural pregnancy. The major contribution of blighted ova to the losses was a feature of all the treatments including those where ovulation stimulation had not been employed but was greatest in the IVF group. In a blighted ovum a fetal pole is not identified in the pregnancy sac on ultrasound; it is the more severe of the forms of disruption which might be identified in clinical pregnancies. It is understandable that it might occur more often in the only group involving embryo handling and potential damage. The chance of fertility treatment pregnancy delivering at 20 weeks or beyond ranged from 67% for GIFT to 75% for the unstimulated cycles.

Table 2 The outcome of Oxford IVF pregnancies (4.87-9.89 1011 cycles) showing results for non-Analogue cycles and Analogue controlled cycles.

	Analogue		Non-analogue	
cycles	762		249	
pregnant	199	26%	33	13%
ectopic	3	1.5%	1	3.0%
TOP (FA)	1	0.4%		
abortion				
6-12 wk	23	11.6%	4	12.1%
13-19 wk	4	2.0%	0	
20-25 wk	5	2.5%	1	3.0%
26-42 wk	163	81.9%	27	81.9%

The Oxford statistics are shown in Table 2. The spontaneous abortion rate was 15.5% and 13.0% below 14 weeks. In view of the current interest in the role of LH elevation in abortion (Howles et al, 1986) the rate was compared with the rate in the non-analogue controlled cycles. The abortion rates in the non-analogue cycles were not different whether considered below 13 weeks or below 20 weeks and an identical percentage of pregnancies reached viability at 26 weeks (Table 2).

Live Birth Rates

The importance of including losses during pregnancy in the statistics available to patients is emphasised by the ILA in the 1989 report. This can give a much more realistic view of what the couple need to know. The difference this can make to statistics can be illustrated from the Oxford figures for the 762 analogue controlled cycles. The overall clinical pregnancy rate per cycle (CP/C) of 26.1% becomes a live birth rate per treatment cycle (LB/C) of 21.5%. The respective rates for primary infertility change from 25.1% to 20.1% and for secondary infertility from 28.8% to 24.5%. The importance of the change is particularly clear when the rates for different age groups are considered (Table 3). It can be seen that the

CP/C is considerably lower for women over 40 years despite there being no difference with advancing age up to that point. As well as the rate of becoming pregnancy being lower, these women over 40 years then experienced a 60% loss rate so that the LB/C was only 2.7% The disproportionate rate of loss meant that although the over 40s had a CP/C which was only 24% of that for women 35 to 39 years old the equivalent relationship for LB/C was even worse at 11.5%.

Table 3 Age and Pregnancy rates in Oxford Analogue cycles.

Age	n	Clin Preg Rate	Live Birth Rate
< 30	129	26.4%	23.3%
30 - 34	301	29.9%	24.3%
35 - 39	251	27.9%	23.5%
40 -	75	6.7%	2.7%
all	756	26.1%	21.5%

Since couples wish to know the effect of repeated treatment we can provide a cumulative pregnancy rate figure with correction for losses during pregnancy. Again this pushes down the figures but is the most realistic guide to the effect of a sustained IVF effort over a few cycles. Even with this downward pressure a couple can be informed that there is a live birth rate of 23.4% for all couples having a first cycle and a cumulative live birth rate per cycle of 50.8% by three cycles (Table 4).

Table 4 Cumulative pregnancy rates in Oxford Analogue cycles.

Pregnancy	try	n	clin. n.	preg. rate	cum. rate
Clinical pregnancy	1	518	142	27.4%	27.4%
	2	152	45	22.8%	44.0%
	3	32	12	27.3%	59.0%
Birth (> 19 wk)	1	518	121	23.4%	23.4%
	2	152	33	16.8%	36.3%
	3	32	10	22.7%	50.8%

Multiple Pregnancy

Since the early years of IVF it has been clear that optimal pregnancy rates result from multiple embryo transfer but this has important paediatric and social consequences so that most centres agree that the transfer of three embryos should not normally be exceeded. As far back as the World Collaborative report in 1985 (Seppala 1985) the twin rate was 10.9% and the triplet rate 2.3%. Since then stimulation regimes and oocyte collection methods have improved so it is likely that embryo yields have improved and the rates of three embryo transfer are higher than in 1985 with a likely increase in multiple pregnancy rates. By the time of the report on the first thousand Bourn Hall babies, the twin rate was 17.6% and the triplet rate 3.9% (Rainsbury et al, 1989a). Recent experience from the Oxford analogue cycles live births, the proportions were twins 31.7% and triplets 3.7%.

Pre-term Labour

Delivery of a baby or babies before 37 completed weeks may constitute a risk both in terms of perinatal mobidity and mortality as well as a higher chance of an operative delivery. The prematurity rate is well known to be higher in multiple pregnancy and is the principal reason for the higher perinatal mortality of multiple pregnancies over singletons. In the Australia and New Zealand collaborative report on 1510 pregnancies (Lancaster, 1989) the observed premature delivery rates were 18.5% for singletons and 56.4% for multiples. Compared with a general population, the premature delivery rate is elevated even for singletons. This effect is again observed in the Bourn Hall statistics (Rainsbury et al, 1989b) with singleton, twin and triplet premature delivery rates at 24.0%, 28.1% and 70.0%.

One difficulty is that of classification of cases which might be categorised as late abortions (20 weeks or more) or as early neonatal deaths. Delivery between 20 and 23 weeks invariably leads to fetal death and at 24 to 25 weeks usually does so. However, in some statistics, some cases might be classified as neonatal death if the fetus appeared to show signs of life and was above 500g whilst in other statistics it could be classified as a late abortion. Accurate details about the classification of such deliveries in IVF pregnancies is difficult to obtain since these mothers are particularly distressed by the outcome.

In the Oxford statistics, as presented in this paper, deliveries of 20 to 25 weeks are shown separately from later preterm deliveries. On this basis the Oxford preterm delivery rates (20 to 36 weeks inclusive) were 8.9%, 28.8% and 100% for the three groups respectively. Similarly using weight below 2,000g which is the weight below which the need for special neonatal care is likely the percentages for singletons, twins and triplets were 6.7%, 31.4% and 76.1% for all cases reaching 20 weeks. By comparison the Oxford statistics for all pregnancies above 500g (1987) gives the rate of delivery below 2,000g as 3.4% based on 5,469 cases.

An important factor which keeps IVF pregnancies from having a higher perinatal mortality is the level of neonatal expertise now available in many centres. For our own neonatal centre at the John Radcliffe Hospital in Oxford the survival of preterm infants is high if born without congenital abnormality (Table 5). The quality of care has been high over many years and the 1987 statistics demonstrate that the preterm infant results continue to improve.

Table 5 Rates of survival of neonates born without congenital abnormalities at the John Radcliffe Hospital, Oxford; 1980-87. (Statistics provided by Dr A. Wilkinson).

	LIVEBORN SURVIVAL		
	1980 - 87	**1980 - 87**	**1987**
Singletons			
500 - 990g	246	61%	73%
1000 - 1499g	447	89%	98%
< 1499g	693	79%	90%
Multiples			
500 - 999g	43	32%	75%
1000 - 1499g	108	95%	100%
< 1499g	151	77%	91%

Analysis of the specific IVF pregnancies reveals delivery between 20 and 25 weeks (little chance of survival) in 4/13 singletons, 2/15 twins and 1/7 triplets for pregnancies delivered between 20 and 36 weeks inclusive. All of these babies were lost whereas for babies born from 26 weeks onwards the only losses were a 27 week singleton after abruption and a third triplet which had a congenital heart defect. For pregnancies reaching 26 weeks spontaneous preterm labour was easily the commonest reason for delivery (4/7 singletons, 13/16 twins and 3/5 triplets).

Another concern has been whether IVF babies suffer an increased rate of major congenital abnormalities. This is not the current experience. In the Bourn Hall series the rate was 2.5%, being 2.0% for singletons and 5.0% for multiples (Rainsbury et al, 1989a). In the Australian series the rate for singletons was 2.2% which was not significantly different from their background population rate. That group have stressed that IVF singletons should perhaps be considered to be a "high risk" group since their singletons had a perinatal mortality of 35.4 per 1,000.

Only time will tell what will be the outcome of further embryo manipulation. An early report on 50 cryopreserved embryos from the French Clamart Unit revealed threatened labour in 20.7% and retroplacental bleeding in 11.4%. There were no congenital abnormalities.

References

Barlow DH, Bromwich P, Walker A, Ross C, Kennedy S, Lopez-Bernal A, Insull M, Egan D, Wiley M and Relph A (1988). Gynecological Endocrinology 2 (suppl 1), 147.

Frydman R, Belaisch-Allart J, Fries N, Hazout A, Glissant A and Testart J (1986). An obstetric assessment of the first 100 births from the in vitro fertilisation program at Clamart, France. Am J Obstet Gynecol; 154: 550-5.

Howles CM, Macnamee MC, Edwards RG, Goswamy R and Steptoe PC (1986). Effect of high tonic levels of luteinising hormone on outcome of in vitro fertilisation. Lancet ii: 521-2.

Interim Licencing Authority for Human in vitro Fertilisation and Embryology (1989). Fourth Report.

Lancaster PAL (1989). Outcome of IVF pregnancy. In Clinical In Vitro Fertilisation ed Wood C and Trounson A. pp 81-94 Springer Verlag, London.

Rainsbury P, Edwards RG, Addo S, Macnamee M, Brinsden PR. (1989a). Observations on the obstetric and paediatric outcome of 1000 babies resulting from IVF at Bourn Hall. Abstract 63, World Congress of Fertility and Sterility, 1989.

Rainsbury P, Edwards RG, Addo S, Macnamee M, Williams G (1989b). "Bourn Babies" - Reproductive outcomes resulting from IVF treatment at Bourn Hall. Abstract 62, World Congress of Fertility and Sterility, 1989.

Seppala M, (1985) The world collaborative report on in vitro fertilisation and embryo replacement: current state of the art in January 1984. Ann N Y Acad Sci 442; 558-63.

Yovich JL and Matson PL (1988) Early pregnancy wastage after gamete manipulation. Br J Obstet Gynaecol; 95: 1120-7.

CHILDREN CONCEIVED BY IN VITRO FERTILIZATION

Introduction

Collaborative studies on the outcome in pregnancies resulting from in vitro fertilization (IVF) have suggested a higher incidence of low birthweight infants, higher order births, and congenital anomalies (Australia IVF Group, 1985; Fertility Society of Australia, 1987; Lancaster, 1987). The higher order births include twins, triplets and quadruplets. The incidence of the preterm births was more than 3 times higher than that in the general population (Australia IVF Group, 1985) and low birthweight infants were predominantly the result of multiple conceptions. The 1979-85 register of IVF pregnancies in Australia and New Zealand has shown a prevalence of major congenital malformations of 2.5% while the national incidence during the same period was 1.5% (Fertility Society of Australia, 1987). The types of major malformations included congenital heart disease associated with transposition of the great vessels and spina bifida. In addition the subsequent development of children conceived by IVF has also been reported (Munshin et al, 1986; Yovich et al, 1986; Morin et al, 1989). One such study which compared IVF with non-IVF children from the general population showed no evidence of developmental delay or an increase in congenital malformations in those conceived by IVF (Morin et al, 1989).

Since 1984 we have followed up children conceived by IVF at St Mary's Hospital, Manchester (D'Souza et al, 1989). In the present study we have assessed differences between children from singleton and higher order births in relation to antenatal conditions, neonatal complications, congenital anomalies, and later outcome since there is much concern about a higher incidence of low birthweight in the latter group of children.

Methods

A total of 86 children conceived by IVF at St Mary's Hospital, Manchester, from 1984 onwards were included. The children were from singleton or higher order births. The mothers received antenatal care at a hospital near their place of residence. Subsequently, the children were seen at out-patient clinics at our hospital. Data on mode of delivery, birthweight and neonatal conditions were obtained prospectively.

Follow up

At visits to Out-Patient clinics height, weight and occipito-frontal head circumstances (OFC) were measured in each child. A general medical and detailed neurological examination was carried out. Details of congenital anomalies were recorded. If a visual or hearing defect was suspected the child was referred to the departments of ophthalmology or audiology for detailed assessment. Development was assessed using the Griffith's Mental Development Scales (Griffiths, 1976).

Statistics

Students t test, or the chi-squared test were used as appropriate.

Results

Table 1 shows that there were 45 singleton births and 18 higher order births which consisted of 14 twins, 3 triplets and 1 quadruplet.

Table I Children conceived by in vitro fertilization.

Pregnancy		Births (Infants)	% Births
Singleton		45 (45)	71
Multiple:	Twins	14 (28)	22
	Triplets	3 (9)	6
	Quadruplets	1 (4)	1
Total		63 (86)	100

Caesarean section rate, preterm births, and small-for-dates infants:

The overall caesaerean section rate was high rising from 12(26%) of 45 singleton births to 11(61%) of 18 higher order births (Table II). The caesarean section rate at our hospital during this period was typically 15%. The incidence of preterm births appeared to increase from 9(20%) of 45 singleton infants to 13(32%) of 41 infants from higher order births (Table III), but this difference was not statistically significant. The frequency of preterm births at our hospital is generally 10% for singleton and <50% for higher order births. The distribution of birth weights showed that there were more low birthweight infants from the higher order births. This appeared to be due to some extent to fetal growth retardation. Twenty-two (54%) infants from the higher order births were small-for-dates, with birthweights <10th centile for gestational age (Milner and Richards, 1974), as compared with 2 (5%) infants from singleton births (Table III).

Table II. Mode of delivery

Delivery		Higher Order			
	Single-ton	Twins	Triplets	Quads	All
Normal vertex vaginal	22	5	0	0	5
Forceps	11	0	0	0	0
Forceps/Breech	0	1	0	0	1
Vertex/Breech	0	1	0	0	1
Caesarean Section*	12	7	3	1	11
Total	45	14	3	1	18

Singleton vs higher order births (All) $x^2 = 6.5$; P<0.01

Table III. Newborn infants

	Infants	
	Singleton (n=45)	Higher order (n=41)
Gestational age (wk)		
>37	36	28
34-36	6	8
<34	3	5
Birthweight (gm)*		
>3500	11	1
2500-3499	30	12
2000-2499	1	19
<2000	3	9
Small-for-dates*	2	22
Males	21	18
Females	24	23
Male:Female ratio	0.8	0.8

Singleton vs higher order births   *$x^2 = 35.13$; P<0.0001

Table IV. Neonatal conditions

	Infants	
	Singleton (n = 45)	Higher order (n = 41)
Jaundice	19	18
Jittery	1	1
Patent ductus arteriosus	1	1
Sepsis	1	1
Idiopathic respiratory distress	2	2
Subependymal brain haemorrhage	1	1
Pneumothorax	1	1
Pneumonia	1	1
Bruising	1	0
No. of infants with any one of these conditions	19	18

Neonatal conditions and congenital anomalies

The frequency of neonatal conditions in the singleton infants were similar to that in higher order births (Table IV). Jaundice appeared to occur more frequently than the other conditions in both groups of infants. Details of the congenital anomalies are shown in Table V. These anomalies were mostly seen in singleton infants. Three infants required surgical treatment for hypospadias, undescended tests, and pyloric stenosis.

Table V. Congenital anomalies

	Children	
	Singleton (n = 45)	Higher order (n = 41)
Hypospadias	1	0
Pulmonary stenosis	1	0
Talipes equinovarus	1	0
Undescended testes	1	0
Large pigmented naevus covering the right scapular area	1	0
Pyloric stenosis	1	0
Tongue tie	1	0
Squint	1	0
No. of infants with any one of these conditions	7	0

Later growth and development

In later childhood (19 to 34 months) a greater proportion of children from the higher order births had weights < 10th centile (Tanner and White-

Table VI. Growth in later childhood

	Children	
	Singleton (n = 45)	Higher order (n = 41)
Weight *		
< 10th centile	1	14
10-90th centile	39	26
> 90th centile	5	1
Length		
< 10th centile	5	10
10th-90th centile	37	30
> 90th centile	3	1
Head circumference		
< 10th centile	2	9
10th-90th centile	41	31
> 90th centile	2	1

Singleton vs higher order births $*x^2 = 16.38$; $P < 0.001$

Table VII. Psychological assessments (Griffiths Mental Development Scales: Mean ± SD)

	Children	
	Singleton (n = 45)	Higher order (n = 41)
Chronological age (mth)	25.5 ± 7.9	24.8 ± 5.1
Mental age (mth)	31.5 ± 8.7	26.0 ± 8.1*
Developmental quotient	116.91± 12.6	106.0 æ 10.9
Sub-scales		
Locomotor	121.1 ± 15.2	116.6 ± 13.8
Personal-social	125.2 ± 18.7	111.1 ± 15.0**
Hearing and speech	117.3 ± 18.4	99.0 ± 17.8***
Eye, hand co-ordination	105.5 ± 11.6	99.0 ± 14.2
Performance	113.6 ± 14.4	102.6 ± 15.2*

Singleton vs higher order births; t test; $*P < 0.05$, $**P < 0.01$, $***P < 0.001$

house, 1959) as shown in Table VI. The distribution of length and OFC values were statistically similar, from < 10th centile to > 90th centile (Westrop and Barber, 1956; Tanner and Whitehouse, 1959). At birth 22(54%) infants from the higher order births had their weights < 10th centile (small-for-dates), while in later childhood 14(34%) children from the same group remained < 10th centile for age. The remaining 8 infants had weights > 10th centile due to increased growth rates from birth. In the singleton group only 1 or 2 children remained < 10th centile in weight in later childhood. The developmental assessments in our two groups of children are shown in Table VII. The infants from the higher order births had a lower mean developmenal quotient (DQ) and lower values for various sub-quotients. These infants appeared to be developing at a slower rate than the singleton infants.

Discussion

In the present study we had difficulty including non-IVF controls from the general population for the following reasons. The parents of children previously infertile tended to have higher incomes, were older than average, and many of the births were multiple. Parents of non-IVF babies from the same hospitals that our IVF babies were born would need to be selected to be matched to the above criteria in addition to maternal age, parity and social class. Since it was not possible to obtain such control parents we have used perinatal statistics from our hopsital, growth charts (Westrop and Barber, 1956; Tanner and Whitehouse, 1959) which are widely used in general paediatric practice and the Griffiths Mental Development Scales which are nationally acceptable.

In a previous study (Morin et al, 1989) the outcome in children conceived by IVF including singleton and higher order births were compared with that in control non-IVF children from the general population. The controls were matched for age of children, multiple conceptions, sex, race, and maternal age. Parental education and income were also matched where possible. The results showed that conception by IVF did not carry an increased risk of congenital malformations or developmental delay. In the present study by comparing the outcome in infants from singleton births with that from higher order births we have assessed possible disadvantages in the latter group by using systematic standard evaluations in all clinical examinations.

There appeared to be an excess of congenital anomalies in our infants from singleton births as compared with that from higher order births. There were no major defects associated with congenital heart disease or neural tube disorders which have been reported previously in IVF children (Fertility Society of Australia, 1987). The affected children in our study had less severe disorders, though three of them with hypospadias, undescended testes, and pyloric stenosis eventually required surgical treatment. Previous reports (Australia IVF Group, 1985; Fertility of Australia, 1987; Lancaster, 1987) which showed an increased risk of congential malformation have raised the possibility that fertilization and early embryonic development in an artificial environment may lead to birth defects. It has been suggested that chromosommal aberrations or mutuations induced by procedures generally used in IVF, or fertilization by defective spermatozoa may contribute to congenital anomalies (Biggers, 1981; Morin et al, 1989). None of the infants in our study had congenital anomalies which are generally associated with abnormal chromosomes.

Various neonatal conditions shown in Table IV are known to occur more frequently in preterm infants. In our study, the frequency of these conditions was statistically similar in singleton and higher order births though there was a higher proportion of low birth weight infants, some of whom were preterm, in the latter group. We did not find a significant increase in the frequency of hyaline membrane disease or idiopathic respiratory disease (De La Torre Verduzco et al, 1976), retinopathy of prematurity (Kinsey, 1956), group B streptococcal disease (Paso et al, 1980), or necrotizing enterocolitis (Samm et al, 1986) which have previously been reported in newborn infants from higher order births.

Initial postnatal growth rates previously studied in twins were shown to be more rapid than that in singleton infants (Chamberlain and Davey, 1975). As a result twins tend to progressively attain a higher weight for age centile over the first two years. In the present study we found that two thirds (n = 14) of the small-for-dates infants from higher order births continued to grow along a trajectory immediately below and parallel to the 10th centile. The remaining third of these infants (n = 8) had attained a higher weight for age centile suggesting an increased growth rate. By contrast, in the singleton group 1 of 2 small-for-dates infants had moved to a higher weight for age centile at follow-up. Similar comparisons could not be made for length or OFC since these measurements had not been routinely carried out at birth. Thus, most small-for-dates infants from higher order births in our study did not appear to increase their postnatal growth rates.

The results of our assessment by the Griffiths Mental Development Scales suggest that children from singleton births had shown better progress in their development than those from higher order births. Two previous studies (Munshin et al, 1986; Yovich et al, 1986), assuming an average developmental score of 100 have reported above average scores for children conceived by IVF. The Griffiths Mental Development Scales or Bayley Scales were used in these assessments. A further study (Morin et al, 1989) using the Bayley Scales has shown that the Mental Development Index Score and the Psychomotor Development Index Score in IVF and non IVF children were statistically similar. In our study the observed differences in developmental scores between singleton children and those from higher order births may bear some relationship to the postnatal environment. We have no reason to think that the extent to which children from singleton or higher order births were 'wanted' were different, or that the personality of parents from the two groups differed in some way. Nevertheless, caring for infants is time consuming and exhausting and attempts to satisfy the needs of two or more children from higher order births may stretch the ability for parenting to the limits of their capacity (Goshen-Gottstein, 1980). Indeed, the lower developmental scores in twins, triplets and quadruplets in our study may reflect the reduced level of parental attention given to these children as compared with that in singleton children.

To those infertile mothers who give birth to healthy infants conceived by IVF and to the obstetricians who assist them the benefit seems enormous. However, we must balance this by documenting the disadvantages of low birthweight and preterm birth usually associated with multiple conceptions. This type of information is therefore vital for the future development of policies for the management of infertility (Wagner and St. Clair, 1989).

References

Australia in vitro fertilisation collaborative group (1985). High incidence of preterm births and early losses in pregnancy after in vitro fertilisation. Br. Med. J., 291, 1160-1163.

Biggers JD (1981). In vitro fertilisation and embryo transfer in human beings. N. Engl. J. Med., 304, 336-341.

Chamberlain R and Davey A (1975). Physical growth in twins, postmature and small-for-dates children. Arch. Dis. Child., 50, 437-442.

De La torre Verduzco R, Rosario R and Rigatto H (1976). Hyaline membrane disease in twins. Am. J. Obstet. Gynecol., 125, 668-671.

D'Souza SW, Rivlin E, Buck P and Lieberman BA (1989). Altered sex ratios. Lancet, ii, 689-690.

Fertility Society of Australia (1987). In vitro fertilisation pregnancies, Australia and New Zealand 1979-85. National Perinatal Statistics Unit, Sidney.

Goshen-Gottstein ER (1980). The mothering of twins, triplets and quadruplets. Psychiatry, 43, 189-204.

Griffiths R (1976). The abilities of babies: a study of mental measurement. Amersham. Association for Research in Infants and Child Development.

Kinsey VE (1956). Retrolental fibroplasia: Co-operative study of retrolental fibroplasia and use of oxygen. Arch. Ophthalmol., 56, 481-536.

Lancaster PAL (1987). Congenital malformations after in vitro fertilisation. Lancet, ii, 1392-1393.

Milner RDG and Richards B (1974). An analysis of birthweight by gestational age of infants born in England and Wales 1967 to 1971. J. Obstet. Gynaecol. Br. Commonw., 81, 956-967.

Morin NC, Wirth FH, Johnson DH, Frank LM, Presburg HJ, Van de Water VL, Chee EM and Mills JL (1989). Congenital malformations and psychosocial development in children conceived by in vitro fertilisation. J. Pediatr., 115, 222-227.

Munshin DN, Barreda-Hanson MC and Spensley JC (1986). In vitro fertilization children: early psychosocial development. J. In Vitro Fert. Embryo Transfer,3, 247-252.

Paso MA, Khare S and Dillon HC (1980). Twin pregnancies: Incidence of group B streptococcal colonization and disease. J. Pediatr., 97, 635-637.

Samm M, Curtis-Cohen M, Keller M and Chawla H (1986). Necrotizing enterocolitis in infants from multiple gestation. Am. J. Dis. Child., 140, 937-939.

Tanner JM and Whitehouse RH (1959). Standards for height and weight of British children from birth to maturity. Lancet, ii, 1086-1088.

Wagner MG and St. Clair PA (1989). Are in vitro fertilisation and embryo transfer of benefit to all? Lancet, ii, 1027-1030.

Westrop CK and Barber CR (1956). Growth of the skull in young children. Part I: standards of head circumference. J. Neurol. Neurosurg. Psychiatry, 19, 52-54.

Yovich JL, Parry TS, French NP and Grauaug AA (1986). Developmental assessment of twenty in vitro fertilisation (IVF) infants at their first birthday. J. In Vitro Fert. Embryo Transfer. 3, 253-257.

A FLEXIBLE APPROACH TO ASSISTED CONCEPTION

During this brief presentation, I wish to bring to your attention two aspects of assisted conception treatment which require further discussion:

A. What is the ideal treatment method?

B. How many oocytes/embryos should be transferred to optimise the prospect of achieving a singleton pregnancy?

What is the optimal method of assisted conception treatment?

One of the main determining factors influencing the method of treatment concerns whether there is functional patency in at least one Fallopian tube. Before the introduction of GIFT, IVF became accepted as a primary treatment option since this proved evidence of the fertilizing competence of gametes besides providing a prospect of pregnancy. Despite the introduction of GIFT, many fertility specialists would commend the fertility management strategy outlined in Table 1 as being the most logical way of conducting fertility treatment in continuity in any given couple.

Table 1. Plan of assisted conception management.

	Blocked tubes	Open tubes
First option	IVF	IVF
Subsequent management	IVF	AI, GIFT etc.

However, since GIFT has been recommended by some as a primary treatment method for those with patent tubes, an alternative plan of management has been put forward (Table 2).

Since there is no ideal laboratory test system which will allow one to definitively assess the fertilizing potential of individual oocytes and sperm,

Table 2. Alternative plan of assisted conception management.

	Blocked tubes	Open tubes
First option	IVF	AI, GIFT, etc.
Subsequent management	IVF	AI, GIFT, etc.
Further management	IVF	?

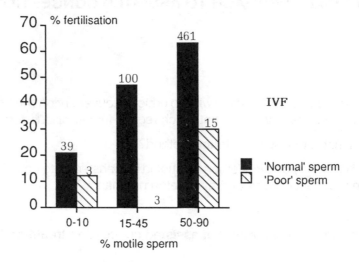

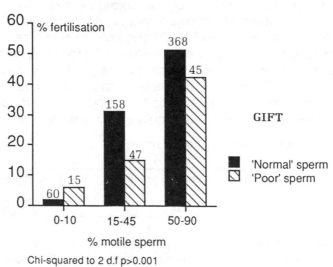

Chi-squared to 2 d.f p>0.001

Fig. 1.
Fertilization Rate Versus Sperm Survival

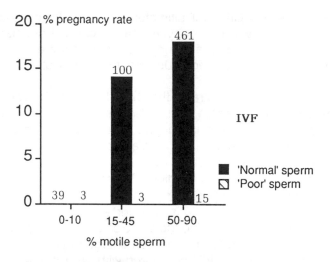

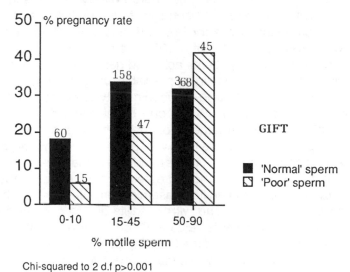

Chi-squared to 2 d.f p>0.001

Fig. 2.
Pregnancy Rate Versus Sperm Survival.

there may be limitations of using GIFT as a primary treatment method in some infertile couples, especially if the quality of oocytes or sperm are considered to be sub-optimal. Whilst the philosophy outlined in Table 1 confirms the fertilizing capacity of gametes, the ability to generate embryos does not allow one to conclude that a particular treatment method, eg, IVF or subsequent GIFT, will ultimately succeed. It is possible that in some couples, fertilization of oocytes may occur in both natural and treatment cycles, and yet pregnancy may not become a reality until another variable is introduced, such as the potential use of donor gametes.

However, we have demonstrated that the GIFT method may have some advantage over IVF in certain circumstances, but it is not possible to precisely identify which individual couples will succeed with this treatment method. Fig. 1 shows the fertilization rate of all oocytes with IVF, and of supernumerary oocytes with GIFT, related to the percentage motility of sperm observed in a culture medium 24 hours after insemination in couples in whom the male partner's semen has been considered to be 'normal' according to W.H.O. criteria, or 'poor' as determined by exhibiting at least one abnormal factor using the same criteria. There is a correlation between the fertilization rate and the percentage motility of sperm. The lower fertilization rate with GIFT, compared with IVF, reflects the fact that the best quality oocytes have been transferred during operation. Fig. 2. shows the pregnancy rates for both IVF and GIFT. Pregnancy did not occur with IVF when motility of < 10% was recorded or if 'poor' sperm was used and yet some patients achieved generation of embryos. However, with GIFT, there was an appreciable pregnancy rate, even with normal semen samples having reduced motility at 24 hours and, in some patients with 'poor' sperm. Whilst one might conclude that GIFT is a preferential method of treatment for men with sperm having reduced motility, or 'poor' semen, there is no way of identifying who will, or will not, achieve a pregnancy by GIFT if this is used as a primary treatment method.

Prospective studies are therefore required to evaluate the relative pregnancy rates for using artificial insemination, GIFT and IVF in patients with unexplained infertility and with infertility due to a specific cause. It would also be of inestimable value if a laboratory test system could be developed which would prove the fertilizing competence of gametes and, in particular, of sperm which would at least lead to a more rational approach as to which treatment option should be considered as primary method.

How Many Oocytes/Embryos Should be Transferred to Maximise the Prospect of Achieving a Singleton Pregnancy?

The Interim Licensing Authority (ILA), Obstetricians and Paediatricians are all agreed that one of the major anxieties about the outcome of assisted conception treatment is the morbidity that accompanies multiple pregnancy. It is on this account that a limitation of a number of eggs/embryos has been promoted to reduce this risk. However, Obstetricians have long accepted that a pelvic scoring system (Bishop) correlates with i) the prospect of pre-term labour occurring, ii) the length of labour and amount of oxytocin required to promote optimum uterine activity, and iii) the probability of a Caesarean section being required. In essence, patients with an unfavourable cervix are more likely to go post-mature, to labour long, to require high doses of oxytocin to promote uterine activity and to require a Caesarean, and vice versa.

With regard to the achievement of successful fertility, it is pertinent to consider that women with fertility problems are a heterogeneous population with different potentials for achieving a successful outcome to fertility treatment which depend on biological and clinical factors and it is my contention that women do not all have the same chance of achieving a pregnancy or having a multiple pregnancy. The risk of a multiple pregnancy relates to a significant degree to:

i) response to drug induction

ii) the number and quality of oocytes/embryos generated and transferred.

iii) the age of the woman producing the oocytes

iv) the quality of sperm.

Evidence in support of this philosophy has been obtained by:

a) evaluating the database of performing 4,000 GIFT procedures.

b) from using two different policies on the number of oocytes for transfer.

Of the population treated, 55% were aged 35 years or more, and 20% of the overall population were over 40 years of age.

The Number and Quality of Oocytes Generated and Transferred

Fig. 3 shows the outcome of treatment related to a number of oocytes transferred in the first 1,357 treatment cycles performed using a flexible policy on the number used (Craft et al, 1988). There is a correlation between pregnancy, as determined by a first trimester scan, and the number used. The incidence of singleton and multiple pregnancy in

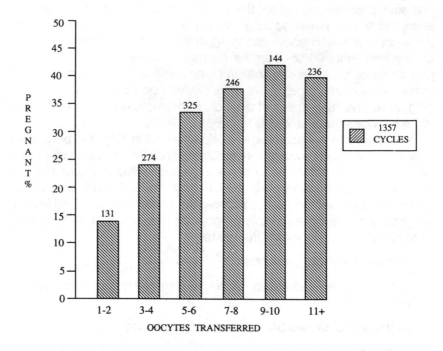

Fig. 3. Outcome of 1357 GIFT Treatment Cycles Related to Number of Oocytes Transferred.

relation to whether 1-4 eggs were transferred, or 5 or more in the 1071 patients having their first treatment is shown in Table 3. The outcome of pregnancy using a flexible policy, as opposed to the subsequent fixed policy, which has now been in force for a considerable period of time, is shown in Table 4.

It is my opinion that women who produce oocytes of different cohort size in relation to drug induction protocols also exhibit different prospects of achieving a successful outcome with treatment. Evidence in support of this view is shown in Table 5 which indicates that if 3, or maximally 4, eggs are transferred from those producing 5 or more, there is an increased chance of pregnancy occurring with the latter group, even though the same number are transferred, ie. 27.2% as opposed to 17.2%.

TABLE 3. Outcome related to the Number of Oocytes Transferred in 1071 Patients Having Their First Treatment.

Oocytes	No. in group	Preg-nant	%	Multiple-Preg-nancy	%	Twins	%	Triplets or greater	%
1 - 4	378	81	21.4	14	17.3	11	13.6	3	3.7
5 +	693	279	40.3	90	32.3	60	21.5	30	10.7
	1071	360	33.6	104	28.9	71	19.7	33	9.2

TABLE 4. Outcome of GIFT Related to Age and Policy Regarding Oocyte Number Transferred.

Age Group	Flexible Policy			Fixed Policy		
	Patients	No. Pregnant	%	Patients	No. Pregnant	%
< 20	0	0	0	2	2	100
20 - 24	21	5	23.8	24	6	25
25 - 29	187	77	41.2	189	47	24.9
30 - 34	414	158	38.2	422	107	25.4
35 - 39	474	152	32.1	406	108	26.6
40 - 44	235	50	21.3	226	38	16.8
45 +	28	1	3.7	26	0	0
All	1359	443	32.6	1295	308	23.8

TABLE 5. Outcome of GIFT Related to Age and the Number of Oocytes Collected with Transfer of a Maximum of Four.

Age Group	1 - 4 Oocytes			> 4 Oocytes		
	Patients	No. Pregnant	%	Patients	No. Pregnant	%
< 20	0	0	0	2	2	100
20 - 24	7	1	14.3	17	5	29.4
25 - 29	30	4	13.3	159	43	27.0
30 - 34	108	24	22.2	314	83	26.4
35 - 39	153	33	21.6	253	75	29.6
40 - 44	121	13	10.7	105	25	23.8
45 +	18	0	0	8	0	0
All	437	75	17.2	858	233	27.2

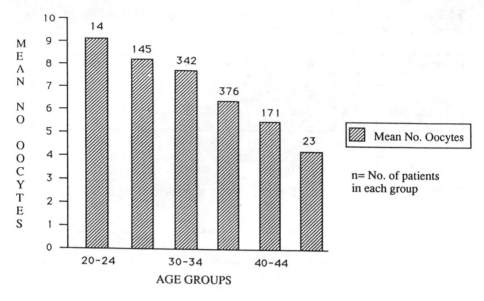

Fig. 4.
Mean Number of Oocytes Collected in 1071 First GIFT Treatment Cycles.

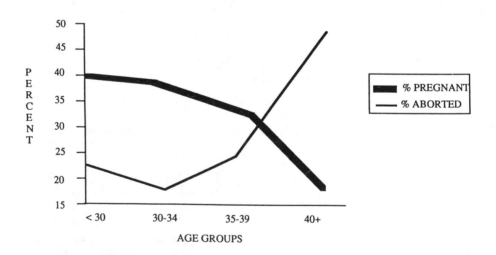

Fig. 5.
Pregnancy and Abortion Rates in 1071 First GIFT Treatment Cycles.

TABLE 6. Outcome of GIFT in 1071 Treatment Cycles. Incidence of Multiple Pregnancy Related to Age.

Age	Total Pregnant	Multiple Pregnancy	% in Group	Triplets or Greater	% in Group
< 30	64	19	29.7	7	10.9
30 - 34	133	40	30.1	15	11.3
35 - 39	126	36	28.6	7	5.6
40 +	37	6	16.2	1	2.7
	360	101	28.0	30	8.3

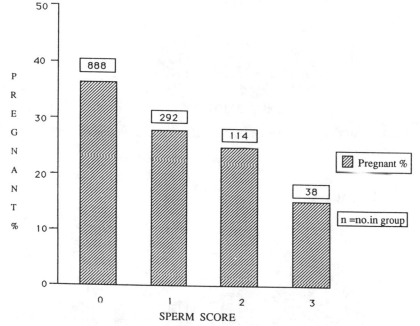

Fig. 6.
Outcome of 1357 GIFT Treatment Cycles Related to Sperm 'Score'

AGE

Women of increasing age produce fewer oocytes in relation to drug induction stimulation (Fig.4). They also exhibit a lower pregnancy rate, especially when 40 years of age or above and a corresponding higher spontaneous abortion rate (Fig. 5). This outcome can be expected even if all of the eggs are transferred into the Fallopian tube. Patients of older age groups also exhibit a lower prospect of achieving a multiple preg-

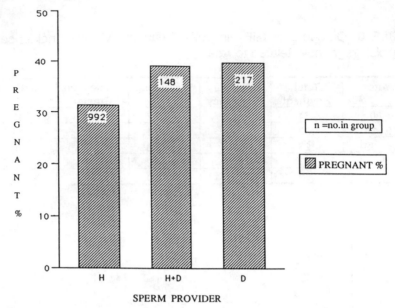

Fig. 7.
Outcome of 1357 GIFT Treatment Cycles Related to Sperm Provider.

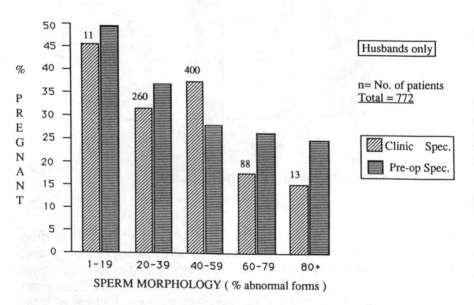

Fig. 8.
Outcome of GIFT Procedures Related to Sperm Parameters.

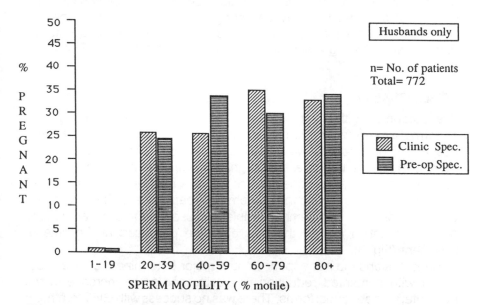

Fig. 9.
Outcome of GIFT Procedures Related to Sperm Parameters.

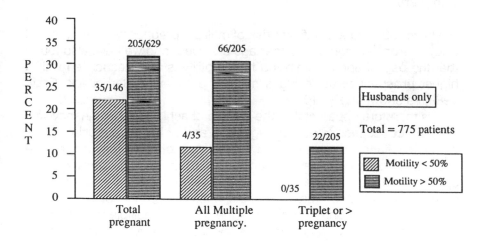

Fig. 10.
Outcome of GIFT Procedures Using Flexible Policy on The Number of Oocytes Transferred. Incidence of Multiple Pregnancy Related to Sperm Motility.

nancy (Table 6). However, we have already shown clear evidence that the biology of reproduction may be changed in older women if donated oocytes from women of younger years are used, since such patients are then at risk of having a significantly higher risk of a multiple pregnancy (Serhal and Craft, 1989).

SPERM QUALITY

The outcome of the first 1,071 GIFT treatment cycles in relation to abnormal sperm factors is shown in Fig. 6 and in relation to whether husband or donor sperm was used is shown in Fig. 7. The more abnormal the sperm factors, the lower the pregnancy rate. The use of donor sperm achieved the highest pregnancy rate, as one might expect. There was also a correlation between the outcome of treatment and the percentage of abnormal forms of a semen sample assessed in the clinic at the time of a consultation and of the split ejaculate produced at the time of treatment (Fig. 8).

Density alone did not appear to be a major determinant unless associated with a marked reduction in motility and/or an increase in the percentage of abnormal forms. There was no success with GIFT treatment when the motility was < 20% in a sample assessed prior to sperm preparation (Fig. 9).

Summary

We have reported a significant risk of multiple pregnancy when donated oocytes from women of younger age are used, and we have also found that the use of sperm exhibiting high motility is also associated with a higher prospect of achieving a multiple pregnancy (Serhal and Craft, 1989) as shown in Fig. 10.

It is therefore apparent that the chance of achieving a pregnancy with assisted conception treatment, eg. GIFT, and of having a multiple pregnancy, is influenced by the age of the patient producing the oocytes, the number of oocytes generated and transferred, and the quality of the sperm (Craft and Brinsden 1989). It is therefore logical to adopt policies of treatment, which will maximise the chance of a pregnancy occurring in individual couples and yet minimise the risk of a multiple pregnancy. A good example of this requirement is the case of oocyte donation where only one or two eggs may be all that is required in a recipient, especially if the husband's sperm count exhibits excellent motility. Similarly, couples in whom the male partner has sperm of sub-optimal quality with low

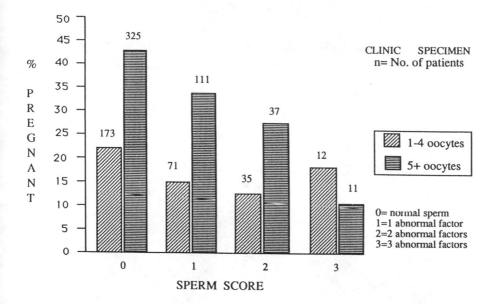

Fig. 11.
Outcome of 1071 First GIFT Cycles - Sperm 'Score' and Oocytes Transferred.

motility may require more oocytes even to achieve a singleton pregnancy (Fig. 11).

These considerations indicate the need for evaluating a predictive fertility score formulated on the lines of the Bishop score, whereby a numerical score, eg 0,1,2,3 would be given to selected biological and clinical criteria. Calculation of a total score for individual couples should allow one to determine how many oocytes (GIFT) or embryos (IVF) should be transferred in individual cases.

There is much to commend a flexible approach to fertility treatment as with every other aspect of clinical medicine.

References

I L Craft, M Ah-Moye, T Al-Shawaf, W Fiamanya, D Robertson, P Serhal, P Shrivastav, E Simons, P R Brinsden (1988). Analysis of 1,071 GIFT procedures - The Case for a Flexible Approach to treatment. Lancet, ii, 1094-1098.

I L Craft, P R Brinsden (1989). Alternatives to IVF: the outcome of 1071 first GIFT procedures. Human Reproduction, 1989, vol 4, supplement pp 29-36.

P Serhal, I L Craft (1989). Oocyte Donation in 61 patients. Lancet, i, 1185-1187.

DEALING WITH FAILURE IN AN ASSISTED REPRODUCTION PROGRAMME

Introduction

Infertility is a major health care problem affecting between 5 and 9% of couples of child-bearing age. The stigma of infertility leads to stress and tension within the family and often leads to marital and sexual problems, mental dis-harmony, divorce and a sense of isolation which is hard to bear. A couple who have experienced infertility and the eventual relief that successful treatment brings wrote in a letter to the Daily Telegraph

> "The sorrow of infertility for a happy couple can be compared with the sorrow of bereavement. The 'funeral' starts when a couple first learns the results of tests which reveal that a problem exists. It continues with surges of hope that a miracle might happen. The sorrow is private, real, and often taboo; failure at any point is always painful."[1]

The sense of failure already exists when a couple present themselves for treatment. They have been reminded of that failure daily as they keep records of temperature and the onset of menstruation is a cruel reminder that yet one more cycle has elapsed without success. They see themselves as being separated from their family and friends who do have children. Our whole society is based on the family unit. Shopping becomes a nightmare when the shops are geared to cater for the baby, the growing child, the school year. They cannot escape the sense of failure, they are left out - they are on their own. They have already failed in their own eyes

---

1   Adapted from a letter from Hugh Henderson to the *Daily Telegraph*, June 6th 1985.

- they are very vulnerable - and this sense of failure can dominate their whole lives.

> "Sometimes I just long to empty my head of all the feelings of hurt, resentment, shame, anger and bitterness that seems to build up inside me."[2]

We all have to cope with failure from time to time in our lives. Often failure is due to something we have done which results in things 'going wrong'. At other times it is because we have failed to do something as effectively or thoroughly as we should have done. We may have failed our driving test, for example, because we pulled out in front of another driver who had the right of way or we failed because we hadn't learnt the highway code. We can see where the fault lies and do something about it before the next attempt. Or it may have been plain bad luck because the examiner was in a bad mood. Whatever the cause it is probable that either we say it was bad luck, and that the chance of that happening again is slight, or we admit the fault and prepare for next time. Failure is transitory, and it is unlikely to dominate our lives. But there will be times when we may have to admit that we are not "very good at some things"; we learn to be realistic in our expectations.

Expectations

Patients who present themselves for treatment for sub-fertility do have very high expectations. Many clinics have found that patients' expectations of success are considerably higher than the success rates which were quoted at their initial consultation. There is a subconscious reluctance to admit that they might very well be among the unsuccessfully treated patients although it is still clear that failure is more likely than success. Headlines in the press "The Miracle Generation", which heralded the 1000th baby born as a result of IVF at Bourn Hall Clinic, raises the expectations of those referred for treatment. A success rate of 15-25% means that the failure rate is 75-85%.

---

2   An extract from a letter in "Child-Chat" #42, The magazine of the support group
     "CHILD", 367 Wandsworth Road, London SW8 2JJ; Telephone 01 740 6605.

Preparation for failure

No one likes to think about failure when embarking on a new venture. There can be very few medical programmes where emotions are so highly charged and where the failure rate consistently exceeds the success rate. It is the duty of all concerned with assisted reproduction programmes to be realistic with themselves and with their patients. Many couples will not be able to cope with the prospect of failure and we should help them to consider the alternatives - including adoption and coming to terms with childlessness. Treatment can fail at many stages - induction of ovulation, oocyte retrieval, fertilization, cleavage, implantation. Failure is potentiated by all that IVF demands of the person - financial, emotional, courage and determination. The Human Fertilisation and Embryology Bill currently before Parliament recognises the need for counselling, and the Government White Paper[3] which preceeded the Bill acknowledges the need for independent counselling:-

"Counselling is a key element in the provision of any infertility service - it is distinct from discussions with a doctor of treatment proposed and should be carried out by somebody different."

Both documents suggest that the prime role of couselling is to prepare couples for the treatment ahead, to discuss all the alternative available (including adoption), to ensure that they understand the implications of treatment with donor gametes and that proper consent has been obtained. But Counselling must go much further than this; it should be a continuing process which starts before treatment is considered, is available throughout and extends beyond clinical contact. Michael Jacobs provides a useful insight into counselling when he says:-

"Counselling does not ignore the obvious, but seeks to reach behind it. It requires the giving of sufficient time to help a person in distress to uncover and reach behind some of the less obvious and less acceptable feelings and thoughts which contribute towards unhappiness and dissatisfaction. It is an approach which has isolated certain factors in caring relationships and stressed

---

3   Human Fertilisation and Embryology: A framework for legislation. Presented by the Secretary of State for Social Services. Cmnd 259, Her Majesty's Stationary Office, London, November 1987.

them, while at the same time played down other factors such as giving answers, expressing sympathy, or actively trying to change the circumstances which appear to contribute towards that distress ... it is above all an approach which tries to understand what goes on inside people, and how internal difficulties can stand in the way of change, rather than looking at external factors or external solutions."[4]

Counselling should be available to help couples through those times of failure and distress. Two of the most traumatic points of failure are failure in fertilization and the return to menstruation which results from a failure in implantation. Couples feel isolated, confused and helpless. Their first reaction is often to ask "what went wrong?", and our reply may have to acknowledge "we may never really know." The idiopathic situation is always the most difficult to bear. Failure is often easier to bear when we can pin point a reason for that failure, if we are expecting it, or if we have been prepared for it. A couple's second reaction may be one of grief, shame, anger or other emotion which may not express itself in words. There is often a very real sense of grief surrounding failure. In grieving a person needs time to lick over their wounds but within the confines of a crowded clinic many will try to suppress their emotions. Anger is often suppressed but comes to the surface in other ways. Sometimes the anger is directed at others because they feel inadequate; often it is directed towards the self - a feeling that you have let somebody down. A man who has just heard that the eggs had not fertilised said "I feel so angry at myself. My wife was the one who had to have all the injections, had to have the operation to recover the eggs - mine was the easy part - now I have let her down, I feel so angry." It may be tempting for the counsellor to shrug-it-off, to sympathise, when what we really need to be doing is to help them resolve their anger, even perhaps confront them with it. It is tempting to hold back when we should speak. Those involved in counselling may be tempted to withdraw when the patient may need that pain to be brough into the open.

A colleague asked me to see a couple who felt that they might not be able to cope with the stres of the IVF programme. They had experienced a series of miscarriages. After listening to them for some time it became clear that they were 'putting on a brave face' for each other. Something I said brought floods of tears to the woman and a very obvious expression

---

4   After Michael Jacobs in "Still Small Voice", SPCK, London 1982.

of hostility from the man which nearly resulted in violence. It was the woman who restrained her husband and then both were able to admit that this was the first time they had allowed their grief to find expression, and that they needed to be able to mourn the loss of those pregnancies.

There will be many times when counsellors feel completely helpless. What can they possibly do or say which will help a person in despair? One reaction is to talk too much in the hope that some 'solution' will present itself. It is perhaps at times like this when one is reminded of the saying "make sure that the brain is operating before engaging the mouth." Just being there with a person in distress, waiting, being prepared to listen, sharing in that helplessness, may often be the best support we can give - waiting together for the anxiety to drop.

Turning failure into success

I want to turn to the difficult question of coping with failure. We have already seen that it is much easier to cope with failure when we can see a definite reason for that failure, or when we see ways in which we can directly influence that situation by our own actions. It is that much more difficult to turn failure into success when circumstances are either beyond our control or where there is no clearly definable reason why, for example, treatment is classed as a failure. Much will depend on our perception of the word failure. That perception may well be very different in those who are supplying the treatment to the patients and in those who are being treated. Those providing treatment in assisted reproduction must be careful not to transfer their perception of failure onto their patients. What may be a disappointment to the clinician/scientist (and which may clearly affect their statistics) may be the starting point where a couple is able to move forward in a positive way even though the starting point is one of failure. It may help to look at some actual cases.

CASE 1

A couple treated by IVF in a private clinic, could only afford one cycle of treatment. Three eggs were retrieved, all three fertilised and showed normal cleavage, and three embryos were replaced. Unfortunately a pregnancy did not result. They were obviously disappointed but some time later phoned to say that at least they knew that **his** sperm had successfully fertilised **her** eggs. They felt that they had done all within their limited financial resources, and they could now accept the situation and concentrate on their love for each other. They felt that they would have been unable to move forward if they hadn't "given it a go."

It would have been very easy to start discussing the 'next moves' with them on day 15 when they had heard the hCG results - to talk to them about the statistical chances of success, that nature on its own only achieves a success rate of 25%, to suggest that it might be worth trying again, and so on ... when what they really needed was time to come to terms with the situation and someone who would **listen** and wish them well. I am sure they would always retain some element of regret, but it was a decision which they could live with.

There is often considerable merit in delaying decisions after experiencing failure. This is particularly so when a couple have just heard the results of a drastic sperm count, or that fertilization has failed; they need time together, to recover from the shock, before even contemplating the next step, particularly if this is likely to involve the use of donor sperm. A deliberate break enables them to talk things through in the privacy of their own surroundings and more often than not they will approach counselling having talked through most of these issues themselves and our task is one of re-assurance and re-enforcement.

CASE 2

A couple who had had 6 IVF treatment cycles, without any signs of success had made a remark in passing "If we are to continue we shall have to sell the house, and buy something smaller, to raise the money for further treatment." It was at this point when I felt that a thorough review of the situation was required and invited them to meet on a Saturday away from the clinic, either in their home or mine. They chose to visit me, and in the event that was a 'lucky' choice.

After reviewing their previous cycles of treatment with them (and previously with a clinical colleague) it seemed to me that perhaps one partner was very much keener to continue with treatment than the other; I was still not sure which was the keener. After struggling for sometime I put it to them quite bluntly "Are you really keen to continue? When was the last time you really talked this over between yourselves? It seems to me that the drive to continue is much stronger in one of you!"

I suggested that I should take our dogs for a walk and leave them together for a while - hence the 'lucky choice' of venue, the dogs played a vital part.

On returning I was met with a smiling couple who put my mind at rest - he had been pressing her to continue because he felt that it was **his** duty to provide the financial resources to make it possible, while **she** was acquiescing because she felt that she should support her husband's 'determination'. Both were relieved to know that the other was fed up with continuing and wanted to "get on with the rest of their lives!".

It would have been very easy to persuade them that there was no reason why they might not eventually be successful - for there was no clinical reason which obviously precluded that option.

We can all quote instances when the reverse would be true; when we have been tempted to suggest that 'enough is enough'; it's becoming an obsession; that surely 'ten' attempts really was enough. Then something inside us (call it helplessness, intuition, a still small voice) made us keep our mouths shut and a healthy baby **was** born in the next cycle.

CASE 3

A couple who had been through several IVF cycles without a pregnancy had asked to have an opportunity to review their situation with a senior clinician and a counsellor. We both spent some time with the couple not knowing what their decision would be. After some months we received these comments from the woman:

> "I have decided not to go ahead with treatment ... since our meetings I have thought hard and long, talking with my husband, family and friends - frequently hopelessly muddled. I believe we have reached a resolution with which I can live ... it is a positive and life-enhancing decision involving a re-committment to my work as a teacher, and a channelling of my energies towards a strength rather than a weakness."

A strong reminder that we often receive strength after having struggled through weakness. It is not often that I use biblical quotations but St Paul in his 2nd Letter to the Corinthians said "I am content with my weakness, and with insults and hardships, persecutions and agonies I go through .. For it is when I am weak that I am strong."

The role of counselling is not to tell patients what to do but to help them process their own emotions by providing them with the time, space and a suitable environment. There are no easy answers, no quick panaceas.

CASE 4

A woman who had been through 4 IVF cycles without a pregnancy, phoned to say that they were not pursuing further treatment. They had found that they would never regret having tried and the experience had brought them closer together. They did not want IVF to dominate their lives and felt that they would try to adopt a baby or toddler who could benefit from the stronger love they now experienced. They did not feel that they had failed at all.

No one can claim credit for decisions such as theirs except to hope that somewhere and sometime during our contacts with them we may have been able to help them to make their own decisions and it does not matter that we are unable to postively make that assertion or not.

On many occasions we may only discover that we have been of some assistance sometime later when a chance remark "I would never have continued if you had not helped me through that terrible time" encourages the counsellor to continue. At other times we will never know. We cannot quantitate it, we cannot judge its cost effectiveness, we will never be able to attach a "productivity figure" against that time we spend in counselling. That should not matter. Common humanity suggests that we do everything in our power to help people in their distress.

9 *B.E. Talansky, H.E. Malter, A. Adler, M. Alikani, A. Berkeley, O. Davis, M. Graf, A. Reing, Z. Rosenwaks, J. Cohen*

LIMITATIONS OF ZONA PELLUCIDA MICROMANIPULATION IN THE HUMAN

Introduction

Human in vitro fertilization (IVF) has progessed from a technique designed to circumvent tubal dysfunction in the female partner to a complex science attempting to address a wide range of infertility problems. As human clinical embryology seeks to alleviate infertility related to gamete interaction, micromanipulation techniques have become powerful tools. When normal fertilization is absent due to abnormalities in the sperm or oocytes, micromanipulation has been used to promote sperm-egg fusion (Malter and Cohen, 1989a; Ng et al, 1990). When polyspermic fertilization occurs, micromanipulation may be used to return the zygote to a genetically normal viable state (Gordon et al, 1989; Malter and Cohen, 1989b). Also, micromanipulation is being used to promote implantation by assisting the hatching process (Cohen et al, 1990a). However, micromanipulation imposes artificial conditions on the gametes. Gaps are created in the zona pellucida. Sperm cells are compressed and possibly damaged in the lumen of sperm injection needles. Enucleation needles enter and disrupt the ooplasmic cytoskeleton. These potentially negative factors must be considered in the development and management of clinical micromanipulation. This chapter will discuss some current micromanipulation results and attempt to address the potential problems.

Micromanipulation to assist sperm-egg infusion

Basic human IVF can be considered a treatment for poor gamete interaction since sperm and eggs are placed in close proximity under carefully optimized conditions (Cohen et al, 1985). Normally, sperm cells must traverse the physical barriers presented by the female reproductive tract. Of the millions of spermatozoa in the ejaculate, only a few will reach the vicinity of the egg. Sperm must penetrate the cumulus cells and bind to species specific receptors on the surface of the zona pellucida. Zona penetration must then occur through acrosome mediated enzymatic digestion accompanied by vigorous tail movement. Finally, the sperm plasma membrane must fuse with the oocyte membrane to begin the process of fertilization. During IVF, an optimum aliquot of sperm is placed in direct proximity with mature oocytes. In many cases this technique produces a high degree of normal fertilization. However, the presence of sperm and possibly oocyte abnormalities as well, often results in a complete failure of fertilization by the most carefully optimized application of the standard technique. Various micromanipulation strategies have been suggested for the promotion of sperm-egg fusion. These fall into three basic categories: the direct injection of a single spermatozoon into the ooplasm; the placement of a single or multiple spermatozoa into the perivitelline space; and the breaching of the zona pellucida to provide an opening through which fertilizing sperm can more easily gain access to the egg. Of these methods, only the second two have been applied successfully in the human. Direct sperm injection into the ooplasm has produced offspring in rabbits (Hosoi et al, 1988). However, this method is highly traumatic and reports from human application studies would seem to indicate that it is inappropriate for immediate clinical use. Zona micromanipulation and subzonal insertion will now be discussed.

Zona pellucida dissection

Gordon and Talansky (1986) reported that when the zona pellucidae of mouse eggs were partially breached by localized acidic digestion, sperm-egg fusion and fertilization were promoted. When sperm concentration was greatly reduced, "zona drilling" resulted in a marked increase in fertilization as compared with control eggs having intact zona pellucidae. Furthermore, offspring were routinely produced following the transfer of embryos resulting from zona drilling. Fertilization and live offspring were also obtained when zona-drilled oocytes from F1-hybrids were insemi-nated at very low concentrations. Zona-intact control oocytes were rarely penetrated when thse low sperm numbers were used. Zona drilling using random-bred ICR mice was also successful. These mice are normally refractory to in vitro fertilization. Sixty per cent of zona-drilled ICR oocytes were fertilized compared to 1% of the zona-intact controls (Malter and Cohen, unpublished results). Zona drilling was then attempted in the human clinical laboratory. Fertilization was obtained in cases where sperm quality was suboptimal (Gordon et al, 1988). However, to this date, no pregnancies have been established following the transfer of embryos resulting from zona drilling.

When zona drilling was attempted on human eggs which failed fertilization during routine IVF, it was felt that the acidic medium used to digest the zona pellucida was causing unavoidable damage to the oocyte and compromising preimplantation development. Zona drilling with acidic medium was therefore abandoned in the human in favour of a mechanical method termed partial zona dissection (PZD) (Malter and Cohen, 1989a). The PZD protocol involves forcing a sharp microneedle through the zona pellucida to create a slit-like opening. The increased perivitelline space needed for this procedure is obtained by shrinking the oocyte in a sucrose solution. Partial zona dissection is a very simple and non-traumatic procedure. Less than 4% of the oocytes are damaged up to the moment of fertilization.

PZD in cases of extreme male factor

In previous studies (Cohen et al, 1990c) performed in Atlanta, we demonstrated that PZD in male factor patients increases the incidence of fertilization by approximately 20% compared to that of zona-intact control oocytes. However, approximately 30% of the zona-intact fertilized, indicating that some of the selected patients were capable, to some extent, of unassisted zona penetration. Several of those patients had previous failure of fertilization when conventional IVF was performed and at least one of them became pregnant following PZD. Nevertheless, we were interested in establishing a baseline for the application of PZD in patients with severe male factor infertility. The following selection criteria were therefore introduced. Patients were only included in this study if the semen analyses had been consistently abnormal. At least two abnormalities were needed for application of PZD. The cut-off values for oligospermia and asthenospermia have been described previously (Malter and Cohen, 1989a), but the normal value for teratospermia was more strict in the current study. Patients with less than 10% normally shaped spermatozoa were considered teratospermic. Sixteen patients were included in the first trial, 8 of those had previously failed fertilization using conventional IVF techniques (Table I).

Only 2 ongoing singleton pregnancies were established in this group. The fertilization rate in both control and PZD groups was considerably lower than in our previous studies (Cohen et al, 1989; Cohen et al, 1990c), presumably due to differences in selection criteria. Nevertheless, PZD did improve the incidence of replacements considerably.

Table I PZD results of the first 16 male factor patients treated at the Center for Reproductive Medicine and Infertility, Cornell University Medical Centre (1989).

Previous fertilization failure	Incidence of fertilisation		Incidence of replacements		Incidence of pregnancy
	PZD	ZP intact	PZD	ZP intact	
yes	9/44	0/38	5/8	0/8	2/8**
(n = 8)	6/44*		4/8*		
no	7/39	2/10	5/8	1/8	1/8
(n = 8)	6/39*		5/8*		
Total	16/83 (19%)	2/48 (4%)	10/16 (63%)	1/16 (7%)	
	12/83 (15%)*		9/16 (56%)*		

* refers to monospermic fertilization only
** one ongoing pregnancy

PZD in cases of unexplained failure of fertilization

Eight couples were selected with unexplained infertility and unexplained failure of fertilization in a previous IVF cycle (Table II). Fertilization occurred in one of the patient's oocytes in the absence of micromanipulation. However, all patients had fertilization when micromanipulation was performed. Fourteen monospermic embryos were replaced in seven of these patients, but pregnancy was not detected.

Zona pellucida penetration failure and oolemma/sperm fusion

The relationship between abnormal sperm morphology and abnormal penetration of the zona pellucida has been described previously (Kruger et al, 1988). The effect of abnormal sperm morphology on oolemma-sperm fusion is shown below in Table III. For this purpose, 16 patients whose spermatozoa previously failed to penetrate the zona pellucida were selected for PZD. The incidence of gamete fusion following zona opening is clearly dependent on the morphology of the sperm head.

Table II. PZD results of the first 8 patients with normal semen analyses which failed fertilization unexpectedly in a previous IVF cycle.

Fertilization		Replacements	
PZD	**ZP intact**	**PZD**	**ZP intact**
17/34 (50%)	7/19 (37%)**	8/8	1/8
14/34 (41%)*		7/8*	

* monospermy only
**fertilization occurred in one patient only

Table III. Incidence of fertilization (PZD) in 16 patients after initial fertilization failure in a conventional IVF cycle.

% normal forms	incidence of fertilization
< 5%	3/29 (10%)
5 - 10%	5/15 (33%)
> 10%	17/34 (50%)

Subzonal Insertion

Subzonal insertion (SI) refers to the direct placement of spermatozoa into the perivitelline space surrounding the oocyte. This technique involves both a physical and physiological breaching of the zona pellucida, and is therefore considered a more invasive form of micromanipulation than PZD.

The need for SI in clinical IVF is threefold. First, it may be applied to cases in which sperm counts are severely reduced and/or motility is impaired. In such instances, sperm samples are of such poor quality that PZD would be an inefficient method for assisting fertilization. For instance, the success of PZD is largely dependent on the ability of the sperm to "find its way" through the artificially produced gap in the zona pellucida. Thus, severely compromised sperm samples (low motility and/or reduced counts) might not be able to fertilize oocytes whose zonae were subjected to PZD. It might therefore be necessary to implement SI in such cases of severe male factor infertility in which direct placement of sperm in the vicinity of the vitellus is needed to assist fertilization.

Subzonal insertion may also be suitable for those cases in which standard IVF consistently results in polyspermic fertilization. This may be due to an ineffective block to extranumerary sperm penetration at the level of the zona pellucida or to additonal unknown factors. Here, PZD would be inadvisable since it requires large numbers of sperm in the insemination suspension. Thus, SI of very few spermatozoa, or ideally, a single sperm cell might be used to reduce or completely eliminate the chance of polyspermic fertilization. This leads to a third indication for the application of SI. Cases of severe male factor infertility for which PZD yields only polyspermic fertilization may require subzonal insertion of spermatozoa. Since it is virtually impossible to control the number of sperm contacting the oocyte which has been subjected to PZD, it may be necessary to employ a micromanipulation technique in which limited population of sperm are brought into direct contact with the egg.

As we discussed, fertilization may be enhanced by the incorporation of gamete micromanipulation into standard IVF protocols. The usefulness of micromanipulation-assisted fertilization is particularly evident when sperm have compromised counts, motility and/or morphology. In addi-tion, it has been suggested that this type of advanced reproduction technology may be used to circumvent outer oocyte barriers that are, for some reason, refractory to sperm penetration. However, despite the fact that gamete micromanipulation has great potential for increasing the chances for successful gamete interaction, it is not without potential disadvantages and risks. These hazards are inherent to any method which disturbs the structural integrity of the oocyte, and may affect the unfertilized oocyte, the zygote, and the cleaving embryo (Table IV).

Table IV. Possible disadvantages of zona micromanipulation

	before cleavage	after cleavage	during transfer	after transfer
O polyspermy	+			
O non-selective fertilization	+			
O seminal toxins	+	+		
O environmental toxins	+	+	+	+
O manipulation damage	+	+	+	+
O abnormalities of hatching			?	+

Based on Malter and Cohen (1989b) and Cohen et al (1990a and c)

Polyspermy

Any procedure which involves the physical disruption or circumvention of the oocyte's natural protective barrier, or zona pellucida, will leave the egg's plasma membrane susceptible to multiple sperm. This is undesirable since it has been suggested that in the human occyte, it is the zona pellucida and not the plasma membrane which is largely responsible for limiting supernumerary sperm penetration (Gordon et al, 1988b). Opening the zona pellucida, such as in zona drilling or PZD, may jeopardize the eggs' priniciple selective barrier and the oocyte may become fertilized by multiple spermatozoa. This polyspermic state may result in an excessive genetic complement and a non-viable embryo. Potential techniques by which such polyploid embryos may be restored to a "normal" diploid state are currently under investigation (Gordon et al, 1989; Malter and Cohen, 1989b). It is difficult to prevent polyspermy when performing PZD since it is necessary to inseminate the oocyte with as high a sperm concentration as possible. Although this will vary according to the requirements of individual cases, a general risk of PZD is that multiple sperm will enter the gap.

If subzonal insertion is used as an alternative means by which to achieve fertilization, the risks of polyspermy could probably be more easily controlled, since exact sperm numbers are determined by the individual performing micromanipulation. However, this is a complex issue. That is, within a population of sperm, whether from a patient with normal or compromised fertility, apparently "normal" cells may be incapable of completing capacitation and the acrosome reaction. Consequently , such spermatozoa will be unable to fuse with an oocyte. It is necessary to artifically induce capacitation and the acrosome reaction in entire populations of sperm to be used for SI in order to ensure selection of a fertilizable cell. However, even if very low numbers of sperm are inserted into the perivitelline space, there is still no guarantee that polyspermy will be avoided. On the other hand, since subzonal insertion of a single sperm can be an inefficient method of achieving gamete fusion, it will generally be necessary to introduce multiple sperm.

Non-selective fertilization

The selection process which precedes fertilization is equally if not more important than capacitation and acrosome reaction. Although millions of sperm are present at the distal region of the female reproductive tract, only a few of these eventually contact the vitelline membrane.

The outer vestments of the egg such as the follicular cells, cumulus complex and zona pellucida all contribute to the selection process by various biological mechanisms, some of which are poorly understood. By interrupting the contiguity of the zona, we are bypassing the oocyte's natural ability to exert selection on the overwhelming numbers of approaching sperm and are therefore allowing a heterogeneous population of spermatozoa direct access to the oocyte.

The ability to penetrate an oocyte and form a male pronucleus does not prove that a given spermatozoon is genetically fit. The role of the sperm cell is certainly not complete at the moment of fertilization. In fact, it has been shown that in the human embryo, transcription is not initiated until a point between the 4-8 cell stage of development (Tesarik, 1987,1988). Therefore, since the contribution of the paternal genome is not immediately evident, a successful fertilization may not necessarily be predictive of a genetically normal embryo.

Some form of selection for genetically healthy sperm is probably functional at the level of the various oocyte barriers. Since it creates a direct channel to the oolemma, zona micromanipulation by PZD somewhat reduces the oocyte's natural control over sperm selection. However, it has been observed in our laboratory that most spermatozoa in the perivitelline space of PZD oocytes had normal morphology. This possibly indicates that the hole can only be traversed by relatively normal spermatozoa. Subzonal insertion may be more problematic, since the role of the zona pellucida in the selection process is completely bypassed. There is a greater chance for an abnormal sperm to fuse with the egg after SI, since it would be selected from a relatively heterogeneous population. Therefore, not only does natural selection play a more influential role in PZD, but the increased numbers of sperm favour fertilization by a normal sperm.

Environmental toxins

Despite all of the aforementioned risks, fertilization may proceed quite normally after micromanipulation. Thirteen clinical pregnancies were obtained in a recent series of 60 male factor patients which were treated using the PZD protocol (Cohen et al, 1989) at Reproductive Biology Associates in Atlanta. This resulted so far in the birth of nine healthy PZD babies from that particular IVF program and several other pregnancies are still ongoing. However, although it facilitates sperm penetration, the presence of a gap in the zona pellucida may allow passage of extraneous non-reproductive cells and foreign substances. For instance, standard sperm preparation methods may not remove microscopic seminal toxins from the insemination suspension. After PZD is performed, such toxins may enter the oocyte before it is fertilized or even after a sperm has successfuly fused with it. This may be detrimental to normal fertilization and/or cleavage.

Similarly, invasion of toxins through the artifical gap in the zona may occur at any point after early embryonic cleavage. For instance, even after replacement, the manipulated embryo is still susceptible to invasion by any foreign cells present in the uterine environment. The possibility of immune cell invasion through the micromanipulated zona pellucida has been investigated (Cohen et al, 1990b). In order to reduce the possibility of immune cell interaction with the embryo, patients whose oocytes were subjected to micromanipulation received low doses of corticosteroids for 4 days following egg collection. Results demonstrated a significantly higher rate of implantation among those patients receiving corticosteroids and this protocol has become incorporated into several IVF programs in which micromanipulation is performed. The mechanisms by which immune cells, toxins, bacteria or other foreign bodies may disrupt the oocyte and early embryo remain undefined. What we can hypothesize at this time, however, is that the presence of a gap in the zona, whether created by PZD or SI, may interfer with normal embryonic development.

The importance or the embryo replacement procedure

The last step of the IVF laboratory protocol in which embryos are handled is the replacement. Although often considered a trivial, simple and standardized procedure, it is actually a critical factor in the success of IVF. During the replacement, mucus, blood clots, and endometrial epithelium may obliterate the end of the catheter; possibly trapping the embryos. Examination of embryos recovered from the external os following transfer in which the catheter was distorted revealed normal morphology. However, this is only true for zona-intact embryos, for it has become increasingly evident that embryos with gaps in their zonae are quite susceptible to damage during replacement.

It appears as though passage through a narrow catheter, often occluded with mucus or tissue, exerts excessive pressure on the embryo. In the case of a non-manipulated embryo, the solid zona is malleable and can easily withstand environmental perturbations. However, manipulated embryos are less suited to withstand external pressure during the replacement procedure. Transfers of PZD embryos have occasionally resulted in the loss of blastomeres, most likely through the gap in the zona. In one particular study, completely empty zonae were recovered from the replacement catheter in two patients in which the zona pellucidae were micromanipulated shortly before embryo replacement to assist the hatching process. The tips of both catheters were filled with mucus, tissue and blood cells (Fehilly, personal communication).

Several IVF programmes which have incorporated PZD into their procedures have reported poor results. Although the embryos resulting from PZD are usually normal and of good quality, it is distressing that transfer of these embryos often does not result in pregnancy. It is feasible to suggest that the replacement procedure in part may determine the fate of micromanipulated embryos. Specifically, it is the type of catheter employed and the vigour with which the replacement is performed, which seem to be critical factors in the survival and subsequent implantation of micromanipulated embroys.

References

Cohen J, Edwards RG, Fehilly SB, Fishel SB, Hewitt J, Purdy JM, Rowland RF, Steptoe PC, Webster JB (1985). In vitro fertilization: a treatment for male infertility. Fertil. Steril., 43, 422-433.

Cohen J, Malter H, Wright G, Kort H, Massey J and Mitchell D (1989). Partial zona dissection of human oocytes when failure of zona pellucida penetration is anticipated. Hum. Reprod., 4, 435-442.

Cohen J, Elsner C, Kort H, Malter H, Massey J, Mayer MP and Wiemer K (1990a). Impairment of the hatching process following IVF in the human and improvement of implantation by assisting hatching using micromanipulation. Hum. Reprod. 5, 7-13.

Cohen J, Malter H, Elsner C, Kort H, Massey J, Mayer MP (1990b). Immunosuppression supports implantation of zona pellucida dissected human embryos. Fertil. Steril., 53, 662-665.

Gordon JW and Talansky BE (1986). Assisted fertilization by zona drilling : a mouse model for correction of oligospermia. J.Exp.Zool., 239, 347-354.

Gordon JW, Grunfield L, Garrisi GJ, Talansky BE, Richards C and Laufer N (1988). Fertilization of human oocytes by sperm from infertile males after zona pellucida drilling . Fertil. Steril., 50, 68-73.

Gordon JW, Grunfeld L, Garrisi GH, Navot D and Laufer N (1989). Successful microsurgical removal of a pronucleus from triponuclear human zygotes. Fertil. Steril., 52, 367-372.

Hosoi Y, Miyake M, Utsumi K, Iritani A (1988). Development of rabbit occytes after microinjection of spermatozoa. Proc. 11th Int. Congress Anim. Reprod. Artif. Insem., 3-9

Kruger TF, Acosta AA, Simmons KF, Swanson, RJ, Matta JF and Oehninger S (1988). Predictive value of abnormal sperm morphology in in vitro fertilization. Fertil. Steril., 49, 112-117.

Malter HE and Cohen J (1989a). Partial zona dissection of the human occyte: a nontraumatic method using micromanipulation to assist zona pellucida penetration. Fertil. Steril., 51, 139-148.

Ng SC, Bongso A, Sathananthan H and Ratnam SS (1990). Micromanipulation: Its relevance to human in vitro fertilization. Fertil. Steril., 53, 203-219.

Tesarik J (1987). Gene activation in the human embryo developing in vitro. In Feichtinger W and Kemeter P. Future aspects in human in vitro fertilization. Springer-Verlag, Berlin and Heidelberg.

Tesarik J (1988). Developmental control of human preimplantation embryos : a comparative approach. J. In Vitro Fertil. Embryo Transfer, 5, 347-362.

THE USEFULNESS OF IVF, GIFT AND IUI IN THE TREATMENT OF MALE INFERTILITY

Introduction

Much work has been done in the application of current technology to the treatment of infertile couples in which the male partner has semen of reduced quality. The aim of this chapter is to review the use of intrauterine insemination of husband's spermatozoa (IUI), gamete intrafallopian transfer (GIFT) and in vitro fertilization (IVF) in the treatment of male infertility, highlighting the benefits and limitations of these techniques.

Patient Classification

The term 'male factor' covers a wide range of semen anomalies, including abnormalities of spermatozoal motility and morphology. During the work-up of the infertile couple, a complete investigation of the male partner must be done (Jequier, 1988) and an assessment of semen parameters made (Glover, 1988). The accurate classification of the man according to the semen profile is important, as the probability of successful treatment is very different for men of different diagnostic categories.

Unfortunately, many reports in the literature do not classify the patients accurately, and this often leads to confusion when comparing the success rates achieved with the various techniques in different clinics

Patient classification is best done using the methods and definitions recommended by the World Health Organisation (1987), with the main categories of patient being normospermia (no abnormal semen parameters), oligozoospermia (spermatozoal concentration $< 20 \times 10^6$/ml), asthenozoospermia ($< 50\%$ spermatozoa with forward progression), teratozoospermia (< 50% spermatozoa with normal morphology), azoospermia (no spermatozoa in the ejaculate) and aspermia (no ejaculate).

Modes of treatment

Intrauterine insemination

The main reason for IUI is to by-pass the cervical canal and deposit spermatozoa within the female reproductive tract to aid transport to the site of fertilization. This can be done with whole semen, but intrauterine insemination of semen can cause severe cramps in approximately 10% of patients (Allen et al, 1985), although this can be as low in incidence as 1 in 300 cases (Joyce and Vassilopoulos, 1981). Also there is the possible risk of infection by the introduction of non-sterile material into the uterine cavity, but the actual incidence of infections following insemination is extremely low (Allen et al, 1985).

The development of laboratory procedures associated with IVF has meant improved and simplified methods for the preparation of washed motile spermatozoa, with the elimination of prostaglandins and inhibitors of fertilization contained within the seminal fluid and an improvement in the proportion of spermatozoa with good morphology (Leung et, 1984). Consequently, many centres are now using their IVF experience in preparing spermatozoa for IUI (Sher et al, 1984: Yovich and Matson, 1988).

Gamete intrafallopian transfer

The technique of GIFT involves the surgical recovery occytes from pre-ovulatory follicles, and the transfer of occytes and washed spermatozoa directly into the Fallopian tubes either via the fimbrial end of the tube (Asch et al, 1984) or the cervix (Jansen et al, 1988). The gametes are therefore introduced together at the site of fertilization. The major difference between GIFT and IUI is that spermatozoa are deposited higher in the female reproductive tract in the former technique and, perhaps more importantly, that oocytes are assured of being released from the follicle and the pick-up mechanism of the fimbria by-passed.

Fertilization and the nurture of the early embryo takes place in the Fallopian tube after GIFT, and this is thought to be an advantage over IVF (Yovich et al, 1988).

In vitro fertilization

The surgical removal of oocytes from the ovary and the mixing with washed spermatozoa in vitro forms the basis of IVF. Fertilization and the development of the early embryo, usually to the 4-cell stage, therefore takes place outside of the body, and the embryos are transferred into the uterine cavity via the cervical canal.

Fertilization can be clearly confirmed by the observation of pronuclei, and the incidence of polyspermy can also be determined.

IUI and male infertility

There are many reports in the literature describing the use of IUI in cases of male infertility (see Allen et al, 1985). However, an assessment of the efficacy of the treatment is difficult as the various studies are often inconsistent in their patient selection criteria, have limited information available, are performed with inadequate control treatments, and use varying methodology.

The confusion and inconsistencies are well illustrated in the series of letters which appeared in the Lancet as shown in Table I.

Table I The 'Lancet debate' on the value of IUI in cases with a male factor present.

Authors	Diagnostic criteria	Pregs/cycle
Kerin et al (1984)	Semen analysis	8/39 (21%)
Thomas et al (1986)	Semen analysis	0/30 (-)
Irvine et al (1986)	Mucus penetration	0/102 (-)[a]
Yovich & Matson (1986)	Semen analysis	5/66 (8%)[b]
		0/22 (-)[c]
Serhal & Katz (1987)	Mixture	6/33 (18%)
Wardle et al (1987)	Post coital test	0/26 (-)

[a] idiopathic,   [b] oligozoospermia,   [c] asthenospermia

Briefly, the debate on the value of IUI in couples in which the male partner had poor quality semen was started by Kerin et al (1984). However, subsequent contributors gave conflicting results as to the success of IUI, but reported on series of patients treated with different methods and selected according to varying criteria.

An evaluation of IUI in the treatment of a range of underlying disorders was made by Yovich and Matson (1988). They showed that a pregnancy rate of approximately 10% per treatment cycle could be achieved in cases of oligozoospermia, but that very poor results were achieved in cases of asthenozoospermia. Poor results have also been described following the treatment of infertility associated with oligo-asthenospermia (Hughes et al, 1987; Ho et al, 1989) and so spermatozoal motility appears to be an important parameter in determining the success of IUI.

Attempts have been made to improve the efficacy of IUI by modifying techniques. In particular, improved results have been achieved by preparing the spermatozoa with Percoll prior to insemination (Marrs et al, 1988) or by the use of ovarian stimulation in the female partner with clomiphene citrate and human menopausal gonadotrophin (Melis et al, 1987).

GIFT and male infertility

Since first described (Asch et al, 1984), GIFT has been applied to many forms of infertility. When used in cases of male infertility, it is generally agreed that reduced pregnancy rates are achieved when compared with results for couples with idiopathic infertility (Braeckmans et al, 1987; Matson et al, 1987a; Borrero et al, 1988; Cittadini et al 1988; Khan et al, 1988; Wong et al, 1988; Guzick et al, 1989; Rodriguez-Rigau et al, 1989), although good pregnancy rates have been described (Silber, 1989; Wiedemann et al,1989).

An attempt has been made to improve the pregnancy rate in cases of male infertility, by increasing the number of spermatozoa transferred (Matson et al, 1987a) based on the assumption that oligozoospermic men produced ejaculates with a reduced proportion of spermatozoa capable of fertilization (Matson et al, 1986). This modification did give improved results, but nevertheless there were still many couples who did not achieve a pregnancy and in which spermatozoal function was questionable.

The major limitation with GIFT, which also applies to IUI, is that fertilization is not observed directly, and if the female partner fails to conceive after treatment then the fertilizing capacity of the spermatozoa has not been confirmed. Therefore, in an attempt to capitalise on the diagnostic information provided by IVF, insemination in vitro of supernumerary oocytes remaining after the GIFT procedure has been found useful (Quigley et al, 1987; Abdalla et al, 1988). Unfortunately, other workers have not found the failure of these oocytes to fertilize in vitro to indicate impaired spermatozoal function, since pregnancies can readily occur in GIFT cycles in which no fertilization of the supernumerary oocytes is seen (Matson et al, 1987d; McKenna et al, 1988; Wong et al, 1988).

However, the limited value of this diagnostic test may well be related to oocyte quality, particularly being influenced by the regimen of ovarian stimulation used prior to the oocyte recovery (Critchlow et al , 1990).

In order to benefit from both the diagnostic information on spermatozoal function provided by IVF, and the nurture of the early embryo in the native Fallopian tube, a combination of GIFT and IVF techniques has been used. Here, the oocytes are inseminated in vitro and after fertilization has been confirmed, the pronucleate oocytes are transferred into the Fallopian tube. The procedure has been termed zygote intrafallopian transfer. (ZIFT; Devroey et al, 1986) or pronuclear stage transfer (PROST; Matson et al, 1987b), and has been found extremely valuable in the treatment of couples in which there is a male factor present and suspected spermatozoal dysfunction (Yovich et al, 1987; Palmermo et al, 1989).

IVF and male infertility

IVF is ideally indicated in the treatment of infertile couples in which the female partner has blocked tubes. Pre-ovulatory oocytes can then be removed surgically from the ovary, fertilized in vitro and embryos replaced in the uterine cavity. However, it has become apparent that IVF is also useful in the treatment of infertility associated with male factors (Mahadevan et al, 1983; Cohen et al, 1985). Here, the in vitro system is used to bring the gametes together thereby eliminating the need for gamete transport, and the visualisation of the oocytes 16-20 hrs after insemination can confirm whether fertilization has taken place.

The precise value of IVF in helping couples with a male factor to achieve normal fertilization rates is debatable. Whilst some studies have shown fertilization rates for oligozoospermic men to be similar to those achieved with normospermic men (Cohen et al, 1985; Englert et al, 1987; Talbert et al, 1987), the majority of workers have reported a reduced fertilization rate and increased incidence of failed fertilization in the oligozoospermic group (Mahadevan et al, 1983; Yovich and Stanger, 1984; Battin et al, 1985; Van Uem et al, 1985; Matson et al, 1986; Awadalla et al,1987) even though a constant number of spermatozoa were introduced directly to the oocytes.

Interestingly, Matson et al (1989) described two populations of oligozoospermic men in their study, namely those in which no fertilization occurred and those in which the rate of fertilization was similar to a normospermic group. This was concluded from the observation that the overall fertilization rate for the oligozoospermic group was reduced compared to their normospermic counterparts, but that the rates were similar when those cases with no fertilization were excluded, as shown in Table 2. The two sets of oligozoospermic men could not be distinquished from their semen analyses.

The idea that different populations of men with a male factor present exist is very important when considering the therapeutic options available to patients. It is unlikely that men with defective spermatozoa would achieve fertilization, even with repeated treatment cycles of IUI or GIFT, but these men cannot be identified prospectively. This is therefore a powerful argument for introducing some assessment of the fertilizing capacity before enrolling a couple onto a GIFT or IUI programme. Unfortunately, tests such as the heterologous ovum penetration test using zona-free hamster eggs do not appear reliable predictors of fertilization (Matson et al, 1987c) , and so IVF should be considered as a first-line option for these patients either as conventional IVF-ET or PROST/ZIFT. Once fertilization has been confirmed in vitro, then future treatment by either GIFT or IUI would seem reasonable.

Table II The fertilization rate (fertilized/inseminated) of human oocytes (From Matson et al, 1989)

Group	All patients	Failed fertilization excluded
oligozoospermia	15/47 (32%)	15/22 (68%)
normospermia	565/823 (69%)	565/770 (73%)

Future therapeutic options

At the moment, conventional IVF merely increases the chance of fertilization by bringing together the gametes. Nevertheless, many couples will still experience failed fertilization. Treatments are now being described which modulate the fertilization process, by either affecting the spermatozoa with chemical stimulants (Yovich et al, 1988), or by reducing the obstacles to fertilization prsented by the oocyte, using hyaluronidase to remove the cumulus cells (Lavy et al, 1988) or micromanipulation in partial dissection of the zona pellucida (Cohen et al, 1988).

Summary

The use of IUI and GIFT in treating couples with a male factor present will result in some pregnancies. However, the incidence of pregnancy is often reduced, and many women will fail to become pregnant with the fertilizing capacity of the husband's spermatozoa remaining questionable. IVF techniques give an opportunity to assess directly the fertilizing capacity of the spermatozoa and, if fertilization occurs, the chance of pregnancy by the transfer of zygotes or embryos. However, a large proportion of couples will still fail to achieve fertilization, and the likeliest therapeutic options would seem to be chemical stimulation of the spermatozoa or micromanipulation of the oocyte.

References

Abdalla HI, Ahuja KK, Leonard T, Morriss NN (1988). The value of IVF-ET in patients undergoing treatment by the GIFT procedure.Hum. Reprod., 3, 944-947.

Allen NC, Herbert III CM, Maxson WS, Rogers BJ, Diamond MP, Wentz AC (1985).Intrauterine insemination: a critical review. Fertil. Steril., 44, 569-580.

Asch RH, Ellsworth LR, Balmaceda JP, Wong PC (1984). Pregnancy after translaparoscopic gamete intrafallopian transfer. Lancet, ii, 1034.

Awadalla SG, Friedman CI, Schmidt G, Chin NO, Kim MH (1987). In-vitro fertilization and embryo transfer as a treatment for male factor infertility. Fertil. Steril., 47, 807-811.

Battin D, Vargyas JM, Sato F, Brown J, Marrs RP 1985). The correlation between in-vitro fertilization of human oocytes and semen profile. Fertil, Steril., 44, 835-838.

Borrero C, Ord T, Balmaceda JP, Rojas FJ, Asch RH (1988). The GIFT experience : an evaluation of the outcome of 115 cases. Hum. Reprod., 3, 227-230.

Braeckmans P, Devroey P, Camus M, Khan I, Staesson C, Smitz J, Van Waesberghe L, Wisanto A, Van Steirteghem AC (1987).Gamete intra-Fallopian transfer : evaluation of 100 consecutive attempts. Hum. Reprod., 2, 201-205.

Cittadini E, Guastella G, Comparetto G, Gattuccio F, Chianchiano N (1988). IVF/ET and GIFT in andrology. Hum. Reprod. 3, 101-104.

Cohen J, Edwards R, Fehilly C, Fishel S, Hewitt J, Purdy J,Rowland G, Steptoe P, Webster J (1985). In-vitro fertilization: a treatment for male infertility. Fertil. Steril., 43, 422-432.

Cohen J, Malter H, Fehilly C, Wright G, Elsner C, Kort H, Massey J (1988). Implantation of embryos after partial opening of oocyte zona pellucida to facilitate sperm penetration. Lancet, ii, 162.

Critchlow JD, Matson PL, Troup SA, Ibrahim ZHZ, Burslem RW, Buck P, Lieberman BA (1990). Fertilization in vitro of supernumerary oocytes following gamete intrafallopian transfer (GIFT). Hum. Reprod. (in press).

Devroey P, Braeckmans P, Smitz J, Van Waesberghe L, Wisanto A, Van Steirteghem AC (1986). Pregnancy after translaparoscopic zygote intra-Fallopian transfer in a patient with sperm antibodies. Lancet, i, 1329.

Englert Y, Vekemans M, Lejeune B, Van Rysselberge M, Puissant F, Degueldre M, Leroy F (1987). Higher pregnancy rates after in-vitro fertilization and embryo transfer in cases with sperm defects. Fertil. Steril., 48, 254-257.

Glover TD (1988). Semen analysis. In Barratt CLR and Cooke ID(eds), Advances in Clinical Andrology. MTP Press, Lancaster, pp 15-29.

Guzick DS, Balmaceda JP, Ord T, Asch RH (1989). The importance of egg and sperm factors in predicting the likelihood of pregnancy from gamete intrafallopian transfer. Fertil. Steril., 52, 795-800.

Ho PC, Poon IML, Chan SYW, Wang C (1989). Intrauterine insemination is not useful in oligoasthenospermia. Fertil. Steril., 51, 682-684.

Hughes EG, Collins JP, Garner PR (1987). Homologous artificial insemination for oligoasthenospermia: a randomized controlled study comparing intracervical and intrauterine techniques. Fertil. Steril., 48, 278-281.

Irvine DS, Aitken RJ, Lees M, Reid C (1986). Failure of high intrauterine insemination of husband's semen. Lancet, ii, 972-973.

Jansen RPS, Anderson JC, Radonic I, Smit J, Sutherland PD (1988). Pregnancies after ultrasound-guided fallopian insemination with cryopreserved donor semen. Fertil. Steril., 49, 920-925.

Jequier AM (1988). The history and examination of the infertile male. In Barratt CLR and Cooke ID (eds), Advances in Clinical Andrology. MTP Press, Lancaster, pp 1-4.

Joyce D, Vassilopoulos D (1981). Sperm mucus interaction and artifical insemination. Clin. Obstet. Gynaecol., 8, 587-610.

Kerin JFP, Peek J, Warnes GM, Kirby C, Jeffrey R, Matthews CD, Cox LW (1984). Improved conception rate after intrauterine insemination of washed spermatozoa from men with poor quality semen. Lancet, i, 533-535.

Khan I, Camus M, Staesson C, Wisanto A, Devroey P, Van Steirteghem AC (1988). Success rate in gamete intrafallopian transfer using low and high concentrations of washed spermatozoa. Fertil. Steril., 50, 922-927.

Lavy G, Boyers SP, DeCherney AH (1988). Hyaluronidase removal of the cumulus oophorous increases in vitro fertilization. J. In Vitro Fert. Embryo. Transfer, 5, 275-260.

Leung PCS, Hyne RV, Clarke GN, Johnston WIH (1984). A technique for enrichment of motile spermatozoa from oligospermic and asthenospermic patients. Aust. N.Z. J. Obstet. Gynaecol., 24, 210-212.

Mahadevan MM, Trounson AO, Leeton JF (1983). The relationship of tubal blockage, infertility of unknown cause, suspected male infertility and endometriosis to success of in-vitro fertilization and embryo transfer. Fertil. Steril., 40, 755-762.

Marrs RP, Serafini PC, Kerin JF, Batzofin J, Stone BA, Brown J, Wilson L, Quinn P (1988). Methods used to improve gamete efficiency. Ann. N.Y. Acad. Sci., 541, 310-316.

Matson PL, Turner SR, Yovich JM, Tuvik AI, Yovich JL (1986). Oligospermic infertility treated by in vitro fertilisation. Aus. N.Z. J. Obstet. Gynaecol., 26, 84-87.

Matson PL, Blackledge DG, Richardson PA, Turner SR, Yovich JM, Yovich JL (1987a). The role of gamete intrafallopian transfer (GIFT) in the treatment of oligospermic infertility. Fertil. Steril., 48, 608-612.

Matson PL, Blackledge DG, Richardson PA, Turner SR, Yovich JM, Yovich JL (1987b). Pregnancies after pronuclear stage transfer. Med.J.Aus., 146, 60.

Matson PL, Vaid P, Parsons JH, Goswamy R, Collins WP, Pryor JP (1987c). Use of the heterologous ovum penetration test to predict the fertilising capacity of human spermatozoa. Clin.Reprod. Fertil., 5, 5-13.

Matson PL, Yovich JM, Bootsma BD, Spittle JW,Yovich JL (1987d). The in vitro fertilization of supernumerary oocytes in a gamete intrafallopian transfer program. Fertil. Steril., 47, 802-806.

Matson PL, Troup SA, Lowe B, Ibrahim ZHZ, Burslem RW, Lieberman BA (1989). Fertilisation of human oocytes in vitro by spermatozoa from oligozoospermic and normospermic men. Int. J. Androl., 12, 117-123.

McKenna KM, McBain JC, Speirs AL, Jones G, Du Plessis Y, Johnston WIH (1988). The fate of supernumerary oocytes in a gamete intrafallopian transfer (GIFT) program is not predictive of a poor outcome: the effect of oocyte selection. J. In Vitro Fert. Embryo. Transfer, 5, 261-264.

Melis GB, Paoletti AM, Strigini F, Fabris FM, Canale D, Fiorettie P (1987). Pharmacologic induction of multiple follicular development improves the success rate of artificial insemination with husband's semen in couples with male-related or unexplained infertility. Fertil. Steril., 47, 441-445.

Palermo G, Devroey P, Camus M, De Grauwe E, Khan I, Staesson C, Wisanto A, Van Steirteghem AC (1989). Zygote Intra-Fallopian transfer as an alternative treatment for male infertility. Hum. Reprod., 4, 412-415.

Quigley MM, Sokoloski JE, Withers DM, Richards SI, Reis JM (1987). Simultaneous in vitro fertilization and gamete intrafallopian transfer (GIFT). Fertil. Steril., 47, 797-801.

Rodriguez-Rigau LJ, Ayale C, Grunert GM, Woodward RM, Lotze EC, Feste JR, Gibbons W, Smith KD, Steinberger E (1989). Relationship between the results of sperm analysis and GIFT. J. Androl., 10, 141-143.

Serhgal PF, Katz M (1987). Intrauterine insemination. Lancet, ii, 52-53.

Sher G, Knutzen VK, Stratton CJ, Mortakhab MM, Allenson SG (1984). In vitro sperm capacitation and transcervical intrauterine insemination for the treatment of refractory infertility: Phase I. Fertil. Steril., 41, 260-264.

Silber SJ (1989). The relationship of abnormal semen parameters to male fertility. Hum. Reprod., 4, 947-953.

Talbert LM, Hammond MG, Halme J, O'Rand M, Fryer JG, Ekstrom RD (1987). Semen parameters and fertilization of human oocytes in vitro: a multivariable analysis. Fertil. Steril, 48, 270-277.

Thomas EJ, McTighe L, King H, Lenton EA, Harper R, Cooke ID (1986). Failure of high intrauterine insemination of husband's semen. Lancet, ii, 693-694.

Van Uem JFHM, Acosta AA, Swanson RJ, Mayer J, Ackerman S, Burkman LJ, Veeck L, McDowell JS, Bernardus RE, Jones HW Jr. (1985). Male factor evaluation in in-vitro fertilization: Norfolk experience. Fertil. Steril., 44, 375-383.

Wardle PG, McLaughlin E, Sykes JA, Hull MGR (1987). Intrauterine insemination. Lancet, i, 270.

Weidemann R, Noss U, Hepp H (1989). Gamete intra-Fallopian transfer in male sub-fertility. Hum. Reprod. , 4, 408-411.

Wong PC, Ng SC, Hamilton MPR, Anandakumar C, Wong YC, Ratnam SS (1988). Eighty consecutive cases of gamete intra-Fallopian transfer. Hum. Reprod., 3, 231-233.

World Health Organization (1987). Laboratory Manual for the Examination of Semen and Semen-Cervical Mucus Interaction. Cambridge University Press, Cambridge.

Yovich JL, Matson PL (1986). Pregnancy rates after high intrauterine insemination of husband's spermatozoa or gamete intrafallopian transfer. Lancet, ii, 1287.

Yovich JL, Matson PL (1988). The treatment of infertility by the high intrauterine insemination of husband's washed spermatozoa. Hum. Reprod., 3, 939-943.

Yovich JL, Stanger JD (1984). The limitations of in vitro fertilization from males with severe oligospermia and abnormal morphology. J. In Vitro Fert. Embryo Transfer, 1, 172-179.

Yovich JL, Matson PL, Blackledge DG, Turner SR, Richardson PA, Draper R (1987). Pregnancies following pronuclear stage tubal transfer. Fertil. Steril., 48, 851-857.

Yovich JL, Yovich JM, Edirisinghe WR (1988). The relative chance of pregnancy following tubal or uterine transfer procedures. Fertil. Steril., 49, 858-864.

Yovich JM, Edirisinghe WR, Cummins JM, Yovich JL (1988). Preliminary results using pentoxifylline in a pronuclear stage tubal transfer (PROST) program for severe male factor infertility. Fertil. Steril., 50, 179-181.

THE ROLE OF OXYGEN FREE RADICALS IN THE PATHOLOGY OF HUMAN SPERMATOZOA: IMPLICATIONS FOR IVF

Introduction

Male infertility is the primary reason for the failure to conceive in about 25% of childless couples (Hull et al, 1985; Cates et al, 1985). Azoospermia is relatively rare and with the exception of antisperm antibodies which are a significant feature in 10-15% of infertile men the biochemical or physiological lesion responsible for their infertility remains unknown. This ignorance is at least partly responsible for the present lack of effective treatments for male infertility and the haphazard state of its diagnosis. Against this background the realisation that poor sperm function is associated with lipid peroxidation (Jones et al, 1979) and the excess production of free oxygen radicals (Aitken and Clarkson, 1987) in substantial numbers of infertile men is an exciting advance which should lead to improvements in both diagnosis and therapy. In this article I shall first outline the biochemistry of oxygen radicals and of lipid peroxidation in general and then consider in greater detail how these processes occur in spermatozoa in particular and how they might be circumvented in the preparation of sperm for IVF, GIFT or IUI.

Biochemistry of Oxygen Radicals and of Lipid Peroxidation

Chemistry of Oxygen Radicals

Oxygen is familiar as a diatomic gas, dioxygen O_2, that is essential to life as we know it. However oxygen can exist in other forms highly toxic to living cells and against which they have evolved sophisticated defence mechanisms (see Chance et al, 1979). Dioxygen can be reduced to yield successively the superoxide anion, usually written as O_2^-, and the peroxyl anion, O_2^{2-}. Both superoxide and peroxide can accept protons and the peroxyl anion is most familiar in its fully protonated form as hydrogen peroxide (Fig. 1). Whilst superoxide and peroxide are more reactive than dioxygen they remain fairly stable molecules of limited toxicity but they can give rise to unstable radicals and complexes, which are both highly reactive and toxic. The further reduction of peroxide yields a hydroxyl ion together with a hydroxyl radical (See Hill, 1979; Bonnett, 1981; Pryor 1986). The hydroxyl radical is an extremely unstable species which can react with many biochemically important functional groups including ethylenic double bonds notably in unsaturated fatty acids, amino-groups, hydroxy groups, aliphatic carbon chains, aromatic rings and various cations and anions. Often a second free radical is a product of the reaction, and this can initiate further reactions so that a single OH· radical can cause extensive damage through a chain reaction (see Wilson, 1979).

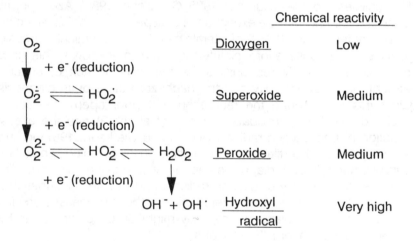

Fig. 1.
The reduction of dioxygen (O₂) to produce oxygen free radicals

Hydroxyl radicals can be formed by the radiolysis of water or by the Harber-Weiss reaction between superoxide and peroxide:

$$O_2 + H_2O_2 \rightarrow O_2 + OH^- + OH^·$$

This reaction is slow but may be catalysed by metal ions. Another potential source of $OH^\cdot$ radicals is the Fenton Reaction which involves the oxidation of ferrous iron by peroxide:

$$Fe^{2+} + H_2O_2 \rightarrow Fe^{3+} + OH^\cdot + OH^-$$

The extent to which these reactions occur in vivo is a matter of debate and it is possible that some of the effects attributed to $OH^\cdot$ may in fact be caused by energetic complexes between superoxide and/or peroxide and iron (see Minotti and Aust, 1989). Another potential toxic mechanism is the reaction between peroxide and chloride ion to yield extremely reactive hypochlorous acid:

$$Cl^- + H_2O_2 \rightarrow HOCl + H_2O$$

Cellular Sources of Superoxide and Peroxide

The principal cellular sources of superoxide and hydrogen peroxide are: (1) The diversion of electrons from the mitochondrial respiratory chain probably at the level of ubiquinone. (2) Oxidase enzymes such as D-amino acid oxidase and xanthine oxidase some of which may be located in special organelles termed peroxisomes and (3) the activity of cytochrome p450 oxidases often located in the endoplasmic reticulum and responsible for the oxidation of xenobiotic molecules (Chance et al, 1979; Paine, 1981). Oxygen radical production by these means is stimulated in the presence of hyperbaric oxygen (see Jamieson, 1986) and of toxic chemicals (see Bridges et al, 1983) and is responsible for at least part of their pathological effects.

Phagocytic white blood cells possess an NADPH oxidase located in the plasma membrane which releases superoxide during the'killing' reaction which occurs when these cells recognise and engulf foreign cells or bacteria,

$$NADPH + 2O_2 \rightarrow 2O_2^- + NADP^+ + H^+$$

The NADPH is generated by glucose 6-phosphate dehydrogenase and the killing reaction is accompanied by increases in the rate of oxygen consumption and glucose metabolism. The NADPH oxidase is a complex of enzymes including a flavo-protein and a special form of cytochrome b and is controlled by a complex regulatory cascade. Its activity can be stimulated by Ca^{++} ionophores, phorbol esters, chemotactic peptides and other chemicals, as well as by phagocytosable particles (see Babior, 1984; Badwey and Karnovsky, 1986; Rossi, 1986; Segal, 1989). The phagocyte NADPH oxidase is strongly inhibited by diphenylene iodonium (Cross and Jones, 1986).

Biochemical Effects of Free Oxygen Radicals: Lipid Peroxidation

Oxygen free radicals can have widespread effects including the oxidation of proteins leading to their degradation (see Wolff et al, 1986) but here only the effect on lipid peroxidation will be considered. An unsaturated fatty acid can react with a hydroxy radical which abstracts a hydrogen atom to leave an organic free radical which can react with dioxygen to produce a peroxide radical which can either continue the chain reaction or react to form a stable peroxide (see Chance et al, 1979; Porter, 1984). The extent of lipid peroxidation can be monitored by following the production of malionaldehyde. The peroxidation of the lipids alters their configuration leading to membrane breakdown and the lipid peroxides are themselves highly toxic giving rise to the oxidation of thiol groups, enzyme inactivation, DNA damage and the formation of ageing pigments (see Jamieson et al, 1986).

Cellular Defences Against Free Oxygen Radicals

Superoxide is converted to hydrogen peroxide and dioxygen by the enzyme superoxide dismutase (SOD):

$$2O_2^- + 2H^+ \rightarrow H_2O_2 + O_2$$

There are 2 principal types of SOD in mammalian cells, a copper/zinc containing enzyme present in the cytosol which is relatively sensitive to inhibition by cyanide and a manganese containing enzyme present in the mitochondria which is insensitive to cyanide (see Chance et al, 1979; Cotgreave et al, 1988).

The principal route for the detoxification of hydrogen peroxide is decomposition to water catalysed by catalase:

$$2H_2O_2 \rightarrow 2H_2O + O_2$$

This enzyme is present at high activity in most mammalian cells but is largely located in the peroxisomes. Hydrogen peroxide can also be reduced by glutathione peroxidase:

$$H_2O_2 + 2GSH \rightarrow GSSG + H_2O$$

$$ROOH + 2GSH \rightarrow GSSG + ROH$$

but this enzyme is more active against organic peroxides and its principal role is probably to reduce lipid peroxides and to neutralise their toxic effects. The glutathione required for this reaction is regenerated by glutathione reductase:

$$GSSG + 2NADPH \rightarrow 2GSH + 2NADP^+$$

The NADPH is produced by glucose 6-phosphate dehydrogenase and the glutathione concentration is a major regulator of its activity.

Non-enzymic methods are also important and cells contain small molecules such as glutathione and ascorbate which can react with free radicals in a chain terminating way as well as antioxidants such as Vitamin E (α-tocopherol) and iron chelating compounds eg. transferrin (see Chance et al, 1979; Cotgreave et al, 1988).

Free Oxygen Radicals and Spermatozoa

The Historical Development of the Topic.

Almost 50 years ago MacLeod (1943) demonstrated that human spermatozoa remained motile for long periods under anaerobic conditions but became immobile in an atmosphere which contained 95% O_2. Catalase could protect the sperm against the effect of O_2 (Table 1). He proposed that the sperm could produce H_2O_2 which inhibited their function and demonstrated that added H_2O_2 had a similar effect. Tosic and Walton (1950) confirmed that H_2O_2 was highly toxic for bull spermatozoa and demonstrated that they could produce H_2O_2 from aromatic L-amino acids present in egg yolk. Seminal plasma could decompose H_2O_2 and protect spermatozoa against its damaging effects. Similar results were obtained by Wales et al (1959).

Table 1 The toxic effect of 95% oxygen on human spermatozoa and the protective effect of catalase (data from MacLeod, 1943). The spermatozoa were washed and suspended in Ringer-phosphate solution pH 7.35, 5% CO_2 was present in all gas mixtures.

Incubation time (h)	% Motile Spermtozoa		
	95%N_2	95%O_2	95%O_2 + Catalase
5	68	10	70
7	60	0	50
8	58	0	53
9	50	0	49

Mammalian spermatozoa are very susceptible to lipid peroxidation and the loss of motility in rabbit spermatozoa during prolonged incubation was directly proportional to the extent of lipid peroxidation (Alvarez and Storey, 1982). Similarly the deliberate promotion of lipid peroxidation in ram spermatozoa by the addition of ascorbate and ferrous ions led to a loss of sperm function commensurate with extent of lipid peroxidation. Lipid peroxidation led to the loss of up to two thirds of lipid phosphate and one half of the content of plasmologen and major unsaturated fatty acids from the spermatozoa. The products are toxic and the addition of exogenous peroxidised fatty acid to the medium caused a rapid and severe loss of sperm function (Jones & Mann, 1973, 1976, 1977a, b). Similar observations were made with human spermatozoa and lipid peroxidation proceeded more rapidly in spermatozoa from men with necrozoospermia than from normal men (Jones et al, 1978; 1979). Seminal plasma or Vitamin E could protect the spermatozoa against lipid peroxidation stimulated by Fe^{2+}/ascorbate and seminal plasma could also protect against added peroxidised fatty acid. Bovine serum albumin could protect the spermatozoa against peroxidised linolenate but not against ascorbate and Fe^{2+} (Table 2). Spermatozoa and seminal plasma from many mammalian species including the human contain superoxide dismutase. Most of the activity in the sperm is easily released eg. by cold shock and is of the cyanide sensitive form containing copper and zinc. However a small amount of cyanide insensitive enzyme is present in sperm mitochondria (Mennella and Jones, 1980).

Table 2 The effect of $125\mu M$−Ascorbate + $25\mu M$-Fe SO_4 or $100\mu M$-linolenic acid peroxide on the motility of washed human spermatozoa incubated for 2h under air at 37°C and the protective effects of seminal plasma, butylated hydroxy toluene (BHT) or bovine serum albumin (BSA) (Data from Jones et al, 1979)

Inhibitor	Protectant	Sperm Motility Index *
None	None	3
Ascorbate + Fe	None	1
	$230\mu M$-BHT	3
	10% seminal plasma	3
	2% BSA	1
Peroxidised linolenate	None	0
	33% seminal plasma	3
	2% BSA	3

* 0, all immotile; 1, 10-20% with weak oscillatory movement; 2, 20-40% with progressive movement; 3, >40% with progressive movement.

lower because of the reaction of H_2O_2 with the cells. Three sources of H_2O_2 were identified, (1) A cytoplasmic system dependent on low molecular weight factors (2) A mitochondrial system stimulated by substrates and sensitive to rotenone (3) A rotenone insensitive system. The spermatozoa contained glutathione peroxidase but not catalase (Holland and Storey, 1981). Rabbit sperm produced malionaldehyde at a linear rate when incubated under aerobic conditions and the loss of motility was directly related to the extent of lipid peroxidation. Lipid peroxidation was more rapid in media with a high potassium content (Alvarez and Storey, 1982). In rabbit sperm H_2O_2 was produced by the breakdown of superoxide O_2^- by superoxide dismutase and O_2^- was presumed to be the primary product of the oxygen radical generation system (Holland et al, 1982). Superoxide dismutase was the principal mechanism to protect rabbit sperm against oxygen radicals (Alvarez & Storey, 1983a). Added taurine, hypotaurine, adrenalin or bovine serum albumin could protect rabbit spermatozoa against autoperoxidation. Taurine penetrated the cells and decreased the production of superoxide (Alvarez & Storey, 1983b). Lipid peroxidation was directly correlated with the loss of membrane integrity as measured by trypan blue exclusion and was associated with a loss of glyceraldehyde 3-phosphate dehydrogenase activity which paralleled the loss of motility (Alvarez and Storey 1984a). Mouse spermatozoa produced free oxygen radicals and underwent lipid peroxidation faster than rabbit spermatozoa and in the mouse glutathione peroxidase was primarily responsible for defending the cells against peroxidative attack (Alvarez and Storey, 1984b). In both mouse and rabbit spermatozoa the rate of lipid peroxidation increased sharply with temperature and the partial pressure of oxygen. This permits the prolonged survival of spermatozoa in the epididymis at a temperature of $32^{o}C$ with a low oxygen tension but means that the lifetime of sperm in the oviduct at $37^{o}C$ and a higher oxygen tension must be limited (Alvarez & Storey, 1985). Human spermatozoa produced superoxide which was partially converted into H_2O_2 by superoxide dismutase. They underwent spontaneous lipid peroxidation and their loss of motility was proportional to its extent (Alvarez et al, 1987). Subsequently it has been shown that the protection mechanism against oxygen toxicity varies between species; rabbit spermatozoa depend almost exclusively on superoxide dismutase and mouse spermatozoa on glutathione peroxidase whereas in human sperm the 2 enzymes are of equal importance (Alvarez & Storey, 1989). Boar spermatozoa are also susceptible to lipid peroxidation but $OH^{\cdot}$ radicals do not seem to be involved in malionaldehyde production in this species (Comaschi et al, 1989).

Lipid peroxidation of the plasma membrane may not be the only site of attack by oxygen radicals on spermatozoa because the motility of de-membranated bull spermatozoa in the presence of ATP survived better in the presence of antioxidants especially glutathione (Lindemann et al, 1988).

In short the early work continued during the 1970s and 80s clearly established that mammalian spermatozoa (including human) could pro-duce superoxide, that lipid peroxidation was a major factor leading to sperm degeneration and that sperm contain enzyme systems to protect themselves against oxygen attack. However the significance of these observations for human infertility was not widely recognised.

Stimulation of Oxygen Radical Production by A23187 and its Pre-valence in Oligozoospermic Men

The current clinical interest in the topic was stimulated when Aitken and Clarkson (1987) observed that spermatozoa from some infertile men produced more oxygen radicals than these from fertile men and that the rate of radical production was stimulated by A23187. They went on to demonstrate that high oxygen free radical production was common in sperm from men with idiopathic oligozoospermia or varicocele but not in normal fertile men or in men treated with sulphasalazine. High oxygen radical production was invariably associated with a poor performance in the hamster egg test (Aitken et al, 1989; Wu et al, 1989) (Table 3).

Table 3. The frequency of different outcomes in the hamster egg test and the production of free oxygen radicals in oligozoospermic and normal fertile men (data from Aitken et al. 1989).

HOPT (% Eggs/penetrated)	Oligozoospermic Men			Normal Fertile Men		
	0-10	11-25	26-100	0-10	11-25	26-100
No. of patients (%)	43(58)	18(24)	13(18)	2(3)	1(1)	70(96)
Luminescence cpm (X 10^{-3}) basal	43	6.3	1.5	5.4	0.3	0.1
+A23187	184	18	3.1	40	1.9	0.4

Free oxygen radical production measured as the luminescence emitted by 0.2mM luminol, A23187 was 50μM and luminescence was measured 3 min. after its addition.

These observations have stimulated further work. Calamera et al (1989) have confirmed that forced lipid peroxidation produces a decrease in zoospermic men after peroxidation. The susceptibility of spermatozoa to lipid peroxidation varied widely between samples and was higher in sperm with poor motility or midpiece defects suggesting that these abnormalities were linked with membrane fragility or defects in the cytoplasmic antiperoxidant systems (Rao et al, 1989). Human seminal plasma contains catalase which is principally derived from the prostate gland and some catalase may be present in the sperm cells themselves. Lower amounts of catalase were present in semen from asthenozoospermic men (Juelin et al, 1989).

Comparison with the White Blood Cell NADPH Oxidase

The oxygen radical production simulated by A23187 was not inhibited by oligomycin, rotenone or antimycin A. The oxygen radicals were scavenged by cytochrome C, a superoxide scavenger, but not dimethyl furan or sodium benzoate or by other scavengers of singlet oxygen or hydroxyl radicals (Aitken and Clarkson, 1987). The enhancable production of oxygen radicals was dependent on NADPH generated by metabolism through the hexose monophosphate shunt (Aitken and Ford, 1988). In susceptible samples oxygen radical production is stimulated by phorbol esters and by chemotactic peptide (N formylmet-leu-phe) and is inhibited by diphenylene iodionium (Fig. 2). The response of sperm preparations to varying doses of A23187 is broadly similar to that of white blood cells but on a cell for cell basis white blood cells produce almost 100 x more radicals than spermatozoa (Fig 3). Therefore the NADPH oxidase responsible for superoxide radical production in human spermatozoa is very similar to that present in phagocytes. White blood cells are a common contaminant of semen and have a deleterious effect on the outcome of the hamster egg test (Rogers, 1986). They are very efficient producers of oxygen radicals and a small (1% or less) contamination of a sperm suspension could account for the observed rate of oxygen radical production. Whilst white blood cells may be responsible for a large part of the oxygen radical production in many sperm suspensions it is possible to make sperm preparations with no detectable contamination which continue to produce oxygen radicals and to respond to A23187 (R.J. Aitken, personal communication) and it remains possible that spermatozoa possess their own NADPH oxidase although definite proof of this remains elusive. A possible physiological role for this enzyme is to increase the adhesiveness of the sperm head membranes to facilitate the initial non specific binding of the sperm to the zona pellucida (Aitken et al, 1989). It is unclear why or how this physiological system proceeds at an uncontrolled and damaging rate in the pathological situation.

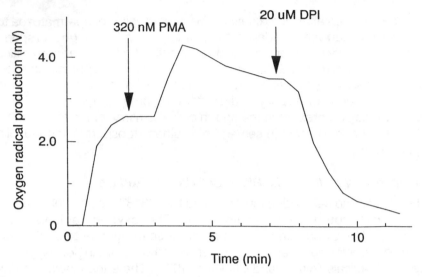

Fig. 2.
A typical experiment to show the effects of phorbol 12-myristate 13-acetate and diphenylene iodonium on oxygen radical production by human spermatozoa. Spermatozoa (9×10^6) were suspended in 0.5 ml BWW medium containing 200μM luminol.Light emission was measured with an LKB luminometer.

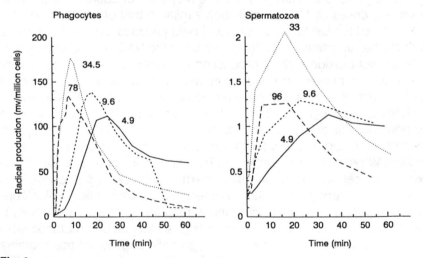

Fig. 3.
The response of white blood cells and of human spermatozoa to different doses of A23187. White blood cells (0.2×10^6) or spermatozoa (3.4×10^6) were suspended in 0.5ml - BWW containing 200μM - luminol and light emission was measured in an LKB luminometer. A23187 was added immediately after the zero time reading.

is unclear why or how this physiological system proceeds at an uncontrolled and damaging rate in the pathological situation.

Sperm Preparation Techniques to Overcome Free Oxygen Radical Production in Crude Sperm Preparations

The objective should be to separate the fertile spermatozoa from the damaged sperm or white blood cells which generate high levels of oxygen radicals and to add anti-oxidants to protect the spermatozoa against lipid peroxidation. Spermatozoa prepared by swim-up from semen, by 'Percoll' gradient or by albumin columns exhibited a higher percentage of motile cells and a greater penetration rate in the hamster egg test than sperm prepared by washing and centrifuging 3x. By contrast spermatozoa prepared by swim-up from a pellet performed worse. This may be because centrifugation into a pellet enhances oxygen radical production (Aitken and Clarkson, 1988). The success of 'Percoll' gradient centrifugation and the swim-up technique rests upon the separation of fertile spermatozoa from oxygen radical producing cells and spermatozoa prepared by these means exhibit a low rate of radical production. The rejected fractions from the Percoll gradient produce large amounts of oxygen radicals and perform badly in the hamster egg test (Fig. 4) (Aitken and Clarkson, 1988). 10mM Vitamin E was effective in reducing lipid peroxidation and enhanced the ability of the spermatozoa to achieve penetrations in the hamster egg test. Butylated hydroxytoluene was a more effective antioxidant but had toxic effects on the spermatozoa (Aitken and Clarkson, 1988; Aitken et al, 1989) (Table 4).

Table 4. The effect of antioxidants on the production of oxygen free radicals, lipid peroxidation and motility of sperm suspensions and the outcome of the hamster egg test (Data from Aitken & Clarkson, 1988, * significantly different from control)

	Control	Butylated hydroxyto-lurene (mM)			Vitamin E (mM)		
		0.1	1	10	0.1	1	10
Post A23187 luminescence cpm x 10^{-3}	47	67	11*	1*	48	39	62
Malionaldehyde formation (pmole/10^8 sperm/h)	9	0*	0*	0*	6.4*	3.8*	2.2*
Motility %	51	45	38	27*	48	48	51
HOPT penetration %	38	31	3*	2*	25	29	50*

Thus an appropriate way to deal with oligozoospermic samples at IVF would be to separate the motile spermatozoa on a'Percoll' gradient and to include 10mM Vitamin E in the media. These precautions should offer a good chance of such samples achieving fertilization of human eggs.

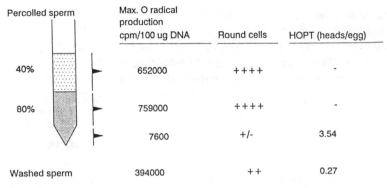

Percolled sperm	Max. O radical production cpm/100 ug DNA	Round cells	HOPT (heads/egg)
40%	652000	+ + + +	-
80%	759000	+ + + +	-
	7600	+/-	3.54
Washed sperm	394000	+ +	0.27

Fig. 4.
The outcome of a typical experiment where a percoll gradient to separate fertile spermatozoa from cells producing large amounts of oxygen radicals was compared to washing the spermatozoa from the same sample by centrifugation 3 times in BWW medium.

Conclusions

Lipid peroxidation is extremely damaging to human spermatozoa and can lead to the complete loss of motility. Slight peroxidation insufficient to affect motility can still prevent them from achieving penetrations in the hamster egg test (Aitken et al, 1989). Lipid peroxidation occurs as a result of chain reactions induced by oxygen radicals. The species responsible may be the hydroxyl radical or complexes of iron and superoxide or peroxide. Human spermatozoa can generate oxygen radicals by a number of routes but the most significant may be a NADPH oxidase similar to that found in phagocytes. The activity of this oxidase is greatest in spermatozoa from infertile oligozoospermic men but it remains to be proven that the enzyme complex is present in the sperm cells themselves and not only in contaminating white blood cells.

Human spermatozoa contain superoxide dismutase and glutathione peroxidase to detoxify oxygen radicals and lipid peroxides and seminal plasma is also rich in radical metabolising enzymes but these protective mechanisms are inadequate when radical production is excessive. The rapid separation on a'Percoll' gradient of fertile spermatozoa from damaged spermatozoa or other radical producing cells and the use of Vitamin

E as an antioxidant in the preparation media offers a good chance of affected samples achieving fertilization in IVF.

Acknowledgements

I wish to thank Dr R J Aitken for introducing me to this topic and for helpful discussions. Work from my own laboratory was supported in part by grants from the MRC and the Birthright Trust and skilled assistance was given by S.C. Harrison, E M McLaughlin, C D Potts and J M Rees. I am also grateful to Prof. M.G.R. Hull for his support and encouragement.

References

Aitken, R.J. and Clarkson, J.S. (1987). Cellular basis of defective sperm function and its association with the genesis of reactive oxygen species by human spermatozoa. J.Reprod. Fert. 81, 459-469.

Aitken, R.J. and Clarkson, J.S. (1988). Significance of reactive oxygen species and antioxidants in defining the efficacy of sperm preparation techniques. J. Androl., 9, 367-376.

Aitken, R.J. and Ford, W.C.L. (1988). Investigation of cellular mechanisms regulating the release of superoxide anion by human spermatozoa. J.Reprod. Fert. Abstract Series, 1,40.

Aitken, R.J., Clarkson, J.S. and Fishel, S. (1989). Generation of reactive oxygen species, lipid peroxidation and human sperm function. Biol. Reprod., 41, 183-197.

Aitken, R.J., Clarkson, R.S., Hargreave, T.B., Irvine, D.S. and Wu, F.C.W. (1989). Analysis of the relationship between defective sperm function and the generation of reactive oxygen species in cases of oligozoospermia. J.Androl. 10, 214-220.

Alvarez J.G. and Storey, B.T. (1982). Spontaneous lipid peroxidation in rabbit epididymal spermatozoa: Its effect on sperm motility. Biol. Reprod., 27, 1102-1108.

Alvarez, J.G. and Storey, B.T. (1983a). Role of superoxide dismutase in protecting rabbit spermatozoa from O_2 toxicity due to lipid peroxidation. Biol. Reprod., 28, 1129-1136.

Alvarez J.G. and Storey B.T. (1983b). Taurine, hypotaurine, epinephrine and albumin inhibit lipid peroxidation in rabbit spermatozoa and protect against loss of motility. Biol. Reprod. 29, 548-555.

Alvarez J.G. and Storey, B.T. (1984b). Assessment of cell damage caused by spontaneous lipid peroxidation in rabbit spermatozoa. Biol. Reprod. 30, 323-331.

Alvarez J.G. and Storey, B.T. (1985). Spontaneous lipid peroxidation in rabbit and mouse epididymal spermatozoa: Dependence of rate on temperature and oxygen concentration. Biol. Reprod. 32, 342-351.

Alvarez J.G., Touchstone, J.C., Blasco, L. and Storey, B.T. (1987). Spontaneous lipid peroxidation and production of hydrogen peroxide and superoxide in human spermatozoa: superoxide dismutase as major enzyme protectant against oxygen toxicity. J. Androl., 8, 338-348.

Alvarez, J.G. and Storey, B.T. (1989). Role of glutathione peroxidase in protecting mammalian spermatozoa from loss of motility caused by spontaneous lipid peroxidation. Gamete Res., 23, 77-90.

Babior, B.M. (1984). Oxidants from phagocytes: Agents of defense and destruction. Blood. 64, 959-966.

Badwey, J.A. and Karnovsky, M.L. (1986). Production of superoxide by phagocytic leucocytes: A paradigm for stimulus - response phenomena. Curr. Topics Cell Reg., 28, 183-208.

Bonnett, R (1981). Oxygen activation and tetrapyrroles. Essays Biochem., 17, 1-51.

Bridges, J.W, Benford D.J. and Hubbard, S.A. (1983). Mechanisms of toxic injury. Annals N.Y. Acad. Sci., 407, 42-63.

Calamera, J.C., Giovenco, P., Quiros, M.C., Brugo, S., Dondero, F and Nicholson, R.F. (1989). Effect of lipid peroxidation upon human spermatic adenosine triphosphate (ATP). Relationship with motility, velocity and linearity of the spermatozoa. Andrologia., 21, 48-55.

Cates, W., Farley, T.M.M. and Rowe, P.J. (1985). Worldwide patterns of infertility: Is Africa different: Lancet, II, 596-598.

Chance, B., Sies, H. and Boveris, A., (1979). Hydroperoxide metabolism in mammalian organs. Physiol. Rev., 59, 527-605.

Comaschi, V., Lindiner, L., Farraggia, G., Gesmundo, N., Colombi, L. and Masotti, L. (1989). An investigation of lipoperoxidation mechanisms in boar spermatozoa. Biochem. Biophys. Res. Commun., 158, 769-775.

Cotgreave, L.A., Moldeus, P. and Orrenius, S (1988). Host biochemical defense mechanisms against peroxidants. Ann. Rev. Pharmacol. Toxicol., 28, 189-212.

Cross, A.R. and Jones, O.T.G. (1986). The effect of the inhibitor diphenylene iodonium on the superoxide-generating system of neutrophils. Specific labelling of a component polypeptide of the oxidase. Biochem. J. 237, 111-116.

Hill, H.A.O. (1979). The chemistry of dioxygen and its reduction products. In Ciba Foundation Symposium 65 (New Series) Oxygen Free Radicals and Tissue Damage. Excepta Medica, Amsterdam pp 5-17.

Holland, M.K. and Storey, B.T., (1981). Oxygen metabolism of mammalian spermatozoa: Generation of hydrogen peroxide by rabbit epididymal spermatozoa. Biochem. J., 198, 273-280.

Holland, M.K., Alvarez, J.G. and Storey B.T. (1982). Production of superoxide and activity of superoxide dismutase in rabbit epididymal spermatozoa. Biol. Reprod., 27, 1109-1118.

Hull, M.G.R., Glazener, C.M.A., Kelly, N.J., Conway, D.I., Foster, P.A., Hinton, R.A., Couson, C., Lambert, P.A., Watt, E.M. and Desai, K.M. (1985). Population study of causes, treatment and outcome of infertility. Br. Med. J. 291, 1693-1697.

Jamieson, D., Chance, B., Cardenas, E. and Boveris, A. (1986). The relation of free radical production to hyperoxia. Ann. Rev. Physiol. 48, 703-719.

Jones, R. and Mann T., (1973). Lipid peroxidation in spermatozoa. Proc. R. Soc. Lond. B., 184, 103-107.

Jones, R. and Mann T. (1976). Lipid peroxides in spermatozoa: formation, role of plasmologen and physiological significance. Proc. R. Soc. Lond. B., 193, 317-333.

Jones, R. and Mann, T. (1977a). Toxicity of exogeneous fatty acid peroxides towards spermatozoa. J. Reprod. Fert., 50, 255-260.

Jones, R. and Mann, T. (1977b). Damage to ram spermatozoa by peroxidation of endogeneous phospholipids. J. Reprod. Fert., 50, 261-268.

Jones, R., Mann, T., and Sherins, R.J. (1978). Adverse effects of peroxidised lipid on human spermatozoa. Proc. R. Soc. Lond. B., 201, 413-417.

Jones, R., Mann, T., and Sherins, R. (1979). Peroxidative breakdown of phospholipids in human spermatozoa, spermicidal properties of fatty acid peroxides and protective action of seminal plasma. Fertil. Steril, 31, 531-537.

Juelin, C., Soufir, J.C., Weber, P., Laval-Martin, D. and Calvayrae, R. (1989). Catalase activity in human spermatozoa and seminal plasma. Gamete Res., 24, 185-196.

Lindemann, C.B., O'Brien, J.A. and Giblin, F.J. (1988). An investigation of the effectiveness of certain anti-oxidants in preserving the motility of reactivated bull sperm models. Biol. Reprod., 38, 114-120.

MacLeod, J. (1943). The role of oxygen in the metabolism and motility of human spermatozoa. Am. J. Physiol., 138, 512-518.

Menella, M.R.F. and Jones R. (1980). Properties of spermatozoal superoxide dismutase and lack of involvement of superoxides in metal ion catalysed lipid peroxidation reactions in semen, Biochem. J., 191, 289-297.

Minotti, G. and Aust, S.D. (1989). The role of iron in oxygen radical mediated lipid peroxidation. Chem. Biol. Interactions, 71, 1-19.

Paine, A.J. (1981). Hepatic cytochrome p450. Essays Biochem., 17, 85-126.

Porter, N.A. (1984). Chemistry of lipid peroxidation. Meth. Enzymol, 105, 273-283.

Pryor, W.A. (1986). Oxy-radicals and related species: Their formation, lifetimes and reactions. Ann. Rev. Physiol, 48, 657-667.

Rao, B., Soufir, J.C., Martin, M. and David, G. (1989). Lipid peroxidation in human spermatozoa as related to midpiece abnormalities and motility. Gamete Res., 24, 127-134.

Rogers, B.J. (1986). Clinical application of the sperm penetration assay (SPA) in locating and diagnosing male infertility. Int. J. Androl. Suppl. 6., 59-75.

Rossi, F. (1986). The O_2^- forming NADPH oxidase of the phagocytes: nature, mechanisms of activation and function. Biochem. Biophys. Acta., 853, 65-89.

Segal, A.W. (1989). The electron transport chain of the microbicidal oxidase of phagocytic cells and its involvement in the molecular pathology of chronic granulomatous disease. Biochem. Soc. Trans., 17, 427-434.

Tosic, J. and Walton, A., (1950). Metabolism of spermatozoa. The formation and elimination of hydrogen peroxide by spermatozoa and effects on motility and survival. Biochem. J, 47, 199-212.

Wales, R.G., White, I.G. and Lamond D.R. (1959). The spermicidal activity of hydrogen peroxide in vitro and in vivo. J. Endocrinol., 18, 236-244.

Wilson, R.L. (1979). Hydroxyl radicals and biological damage in vitro: what relevance in vivo. In: Ciba Foundation Symposium 65 (new series) Oxygen Radicals and Tissue Damage Excerpta Medica, Amsterdam, pp19-42.

Wolff, S.P., Garner, A. and Dean, R.T. (1986). Free radicals, lipids and protein degradation. T.I.B.S., 11, 27-31.

Wu, F.C.W., Aitken, R.J. and Ferguson, A., (1989). Inflammatory bowel disease and male infertility: effects of sulphasalazine and 5- amino salicylic acid on sperm fertilising capacity and reactive oxygen species generation. Fertil. Steril., 52, 842-845.

GONADOTROPHIN THERAPY IN THE MALE

Introduction

The process of sperm production and maturation is started, modulated and accomplished by hormonal mechanisms. By the way, the hormonal treatment of oligozoospermias from tubular failure has been so far unrewarding, mainly due to our incomplete knowledge of the intimate mechanisms of the spermatogenesis, and possibly to improper diagnostic criteria (Isidori, 1981; Eliasson, 1983; Schill, 1986; Isidori, 1988). At present, recent basic and clinical studies have opened new possibilities of improving the sperm production and maturation acting on hormonal mechanisms. Thus, hormones and hormone-like substances can be used, acting through different pathways but reaching the ultimate target of regulating spermatogenesis essentially: a) modulating the pituitary secretory activity (centrally-acting substances); b) acting directly on the testicular tissues (gonadotrophins) and c) modulating the intra-testicular auto-and paracrine mechanisms (see Table I).

Centrally-acting substances

Neurotransmitters and neuromodulators, acting at hypothalamic and/or pituitary levels, have been shown to restore to normal an impaired secretory activity. Thus, the administration of opioidpeptide antagonists (Naloxone or Naltrexone), increases significantly a reduced gonadotrophin secretion due to an excess of opioid peptides as shown in Fig.1.

Table I. Hormonal treatment in tubular failures (oligozoospermias).

Substances	Target
Agonists and/or Antagonists of Neurotransmitters	
Antiestrogens	Hypothalamus
"Rebound"	
GnRH	Pituitary
Gonadotrophins	
(HCG + HMG)	Testis
(FSH)	
Agonists and/or Antagonists of local intratesticular factors	Intratesticular para/auto-crine mechanisms
Androgens	Androgen-sensitive structures

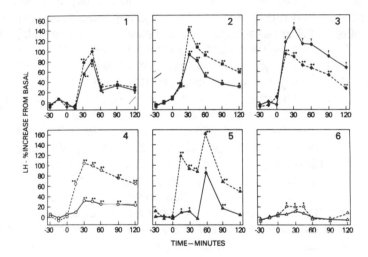

Fig. 1.
The Naloxone test. The i.v. administration of opioid-anatagonist Naloxone i.v. (100 mcg in bolus) increases both RIA (solid lines) and BIO (dotted lines) assayed LH Gonadotrophin levels.

Interesting results are obtained with the pulsatile administration of GnRH in cases of hypothalamic failure, while well known is the effect of the anti-estrogens (Clomiphene, Tamoxiphene) on the hypothalamic-pituitary activity (Eliasson, 1983). These forms of treatment are nevertheless limited to selected cases (Isidori, 1988) namely when a proper diagnosis has been made (for instance, the already quoted excess of opioid peptides or impaired activity of the arcuate nucleus of the hypothalamus; provided that the pituitary gonadotrophs are anatomically and functionally adequate). Furthermore, the use of such compounds should be carefully monitored, due to the possibility of untoward effects of a prolonged administration, as it is necessary in the treatment of the spermatogenetic failures.

Gonadoptrophins (GT)

Criteria of use

The gonadotrophins (FSH and ICSH or LH), are the physiological factors stimulating the spermatogenesis acting through different but co-operating mechanisms and pathways at testicular level. But, so far, only the **quantitative** failures of GT production (ie., low circulating radioimmunoassayed levels of plasma GT in basal conditions and after provocative tests), were considered responsible for defective spermatogenesis and thus eligible for a treatment with exogenous GT. These forms, the Hypogonadotrophic Hypogonadisms (HH), amount to less than 10% of all oligozoospermias. By the way, according to the new endocrinological trends, new cases have been identified in which the GT are quantitatively normal at the RIA, but **biologically ineffective** (Isidori, 1981; Isidori,1988). Table II enlists some of the possible central and peripheral causes of inadequate gonadotrophin activity (IGA),which can be responsible for oligozoospermias, cryptorchidsm, delayed puberty, etc. The diagnostic criteria for detecting a case of IGA are mainly aimed to demonstrate a reduced biological activity of the GT and to rule out a peripheral damage (see Table III). According to these selecting criteria, 25% of cases of oligozoospermias from tubular failure from central defect (HH + IGA so far classified as "idiopathic oligozoospermias") can be treated with exogenous GT as seen in Fig. 2.

Therapeutic protocol

The therapeutic protocol thus adopted in these cases is the following:

HCG: 4000 I.U. as LH weekly and HMG (or pure FSH = METRODIN): 225 I.U. weekly for three months. The HCG can be administered in one single dose, due to the long half-life of the compound, whose effects on the testosterone production last for at least one week; while the FSH, due to the shorter half-life, must be administered in refracted doses. The course can be repeated after a two-months interval. The associated (HCG + HMG or FSH) treatment seems to be more physiological in the oligozoospermias from tubular failure, considering the close co-operation of the two principles inside the testicular structures. By the way, the use of FSH alone can be hypothesized in cases with good interstitial activity. Controlled studies in this concern are in progress.

Table II. Factors influencing gonadotrophin activity.

Site of Activity	Influencing Factors
Central	Neurotransmission
	Neuromodulation
	Pulsatility
	Glycosilation
	Reduced bioactivity of the molecule
	Alpha- or beta- preferential gene activation
Peripheral	Turnover
	Clearance
	Receptor binding
	Transduction
	cAMP activation

Table III. Diagnostic criteria for the admission to the GT treatment.

Assessment	Diagnostic criteria
Inadequate GT secretion	Plasma RIA levels of GT low or normal in basal condition and after provocative tests (100 mcg e.v. in bolus)
	Bioassay of LH and FSH (RICT for LH and GCT for FSH): low B/I ratio
	(Pulsatility studies, Naloxone test, Clomiphene test).
	Prolactin assay
Peripheral damage	Biochemical, structural and immunological study of the seminal fluid.
	Response to the HCG test
	(Testicular hystology)

Results

In cases selected according to the aforementioned criteria, an 85% improvement of spermatogenesis, including the Theoretical Fertility Potential (TFP, see after), has been recorded; with a 37.7% rate of spontaneous pregnancies. The lack of response in 15% of cases can be

UNIVERSITY OF ROME – DEPT. ANDROLOGY

GT TREATMENT: SELECTION OF PATIENTS (%)

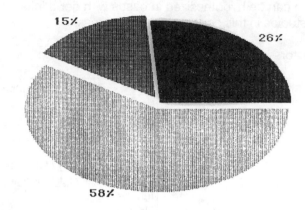

Fig. 2.
Selection of oligospermic patients for the admission to the GT treatment: 15% :
Undiagnosed; 26.1% : Cases admitted to GT treatment (HH + IGA); 58.9% :
"Excretory oligozoospermias".

GT TREATMENT: EFFECTS

85% = spz.incr. 37.7% = preg. rate

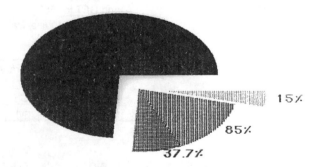

Fig. 3.
Results of the GT treatment in the selected cases : 85% : Improvement of spermatogenesis; 37.7% : Spontaneous pregnancies in this group ; 15%: Failures.

due to a variety of reasons, including inadequate absorption, transport or delivery of the drugs, undiagnosed peripheral defects, etc. With these doses and modality of treatment, no untoward effects (down-regulation of pituitary and/or testicular receptors), overstimulation (thickening of the basement membrane), antibody formation, etc., have significantly been recorded.

Controlled Studies

Six patients with idiopathic oligozoospermia, diagnosed as cases of IGA, were followed for one year prior to the admission to the exogenous GT regimen. They were not treated at all or treated (by us or others), with "supportive" therapy (vitamins, aminoacids, oral testosterone). Their seminal fluids were checked monthly in that pretreatment year and in the following year, when they were submitted to the GT treatment (two courses). Fig. 4 shows clearly the significance of this intra-patient controlled study.

The Theoretical Fertility Potential (TFP)

At present, the classical seminal parameters for the evaluation of the effects of a given treatment (concentration, motility and morphology of the sperms), seem no longer adequate. Actually, the modern procedures for AI and IVF have focused the attention on the intrinsic properties of the

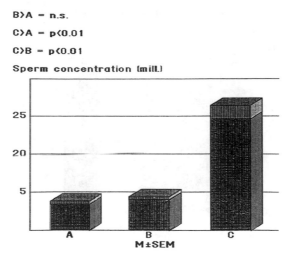

Fig. 4.
Sperm concentration in a group of patients with IGA selected for GT treatment, in basal condition (A), after one year without treatment (B) and after two courses of GT treatment (C) (means on multiple assays: M ± SEM)

single spermatic cells as such, being other properties easily manipulated. Furthermore, it becomes increasingly evident that many of the failures in this procedures are due to intrinsic anomalies of the spermatic cell (Barvin,

Table IV. The Theoretical Fertility Potential of spermatozoa.

Investigation	Tests
Cellular integrity	Membrane LPO (n.v. 8.75-3.30 MDA/10 spz)
	Acrosine (n.v. 10.54-1.16 ng/10spz)
	Chromatin heterogeneity (n.v. 50% of green cells)
	Swelling test (n.v. 50% of swollen cells with 150 mosm/l sol.)
	Seminal LDH-X
	Triple staining
Functional capacity	ATP (n.v. 10-100 ng/10spz)
	Computerized velocimetry
	Penetration tests (Alexander's; Kramer's)

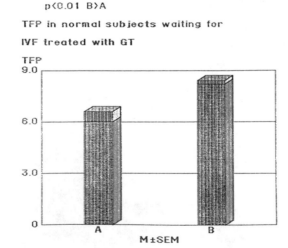

p<0.01 B>A

TFP in normal subjects waiting for

IVF treated with GT

M±SEM

Fig. 5.
Fig 5. TFP (Theoretical Fertility Potential) in normal subjects (10) waiting for an IVF program after short-term, low-dose course of GT treatment (see text). A = TFP in basal conditions; B = after treatment (M ± SEM).

1986). We have therefore proposed a Theoretical Fertility Potential (TFP) index, based upon the results of some tests assessing the integrity and functionality of the spermatic cell (Isidori, 1987), as shown in Table IV. The results of each test is arbitrarily scored 0-0.5-1. The final score ranges therefore from 0 to 10. The higher the score, the higher the probability for the considered spermatozoa to fertilize the ovum. The GT treatment increases the TFP in oligozoospermic patients, as already published (Isidori, 1988); and this gives support to the well known observation that the sperms of hypogonadotrophic patients treated with GT induce pregnancies in very low concentrations, beyond the considered minimum normal. On this basis, in studies still in progress, we have observed that a mild GT treatment (1000 IU of HCG and 150 of FSH weekly for two months), increases the TFP in **normal** subjects waiting for an IVF program for female problems (Fig. 5). This preliminary finding seems particularly worthy of interest in view of the many unexplained failures of IVF procedures, probably due to undetected, intrinsic defects of apparently "normal" sperms. It must be obviously validated with controlled studies comparing the pregnancy rates obtained in these versus non-treated subjects. The TFP improves also in adult, ex-**cryptorchid** subjects treated with GT in childhood, irrespective of the descensus of the testis, which was obtained with surgery. This has been shown in a retrospective study

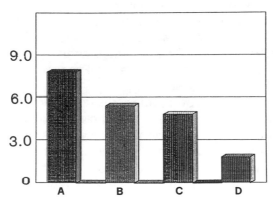

Fig. 6.
TFP in adult, ex-cryptorchid subjects, all operated for orchypexis. From left to right : (A) Monolateral, treated with GT; (B) Monolateral, treated with GT; (B) Monolateral untreated; (C) Bilateral treated; (D) Bilateral untreated.

comparing groups of adults subjects, ex mono- or bilateral cryptorchid, all operated but also treated with GT, versus similar patients operated but not treated (Fig. 6). The improvement of the TFP parallels the increase of sperm concentration, (Isidor et al, 1989) and underlines the problem of the future functionality of the cryptorchid tests even when properly operated.

Substances acting on intratesticular local mechanisms

Recent emphasis has been put on the substances produced and acting inside the testis and regulating - via paracrine and autocrine mechanisms - the cellular activities and the cell-to-cell transmission of the central message (Dufau, 1988; Bellve and Zheng, 1989; Berry and Pescovits, 1989; Fabbri et al, 1989b; Fabbri, 1990). A variety of locally produced "inhibins" and "activins" has been identified, some of them acting both at peripheral and central level; but this is not the place to examine them in detail. By the way, at present clinical interest has been raised by some inhibiting substances (beta-endorphine, CRF) and by some stimulating factors (Growth Factors : GRF, somatomedins, etc.). Beta-endorphine is produced by the Leydig cells and acts on the Sertoli cells reducing sharply the production of ABP (paracrine mechanism). The CRF is produced by the Leydig cells too, increase the production of beta-endorphine and reduces the production of testosterone by an autocrine mechanism (Fabri et al, 1986; Fabbri et al, 1989a; Fabbri et al, 1990). Somatomedin C (SMC = IGF I) is produced by Sertoli cells and increases the production of testosterone by the Leydig cells, enhances the sensitivity of the Sertoli cells to the FSH and has some receptors on the spermatic cells themselves. GRF (Growth-Hormone Releasing-Factor) may act similarly via stimulation of SMC or independantly.

It seems reasonable to overcome some unexplained forms of arrested spermatogenesis (possibly due to an unbalance among the two groups of factors), or by removing inhibiting factors or by enhancing the growth factors. Preliminary results are encouraging (see Fig. 7 and Fig. 8.), although we firmly believe that further, controlled studies are needed to define the biological role and the therapeutic potential of these and similar substances in male infertility.

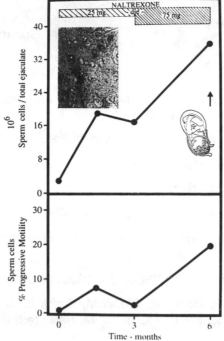

Fig. 7.
Effect of treatment with Naltrexone (25 mg p. os for 3 months and 75 mg p. os for 3 months), on sperm concentration and motility, in an oligospermic subject with high intratesticular amount of beta-endorphine.

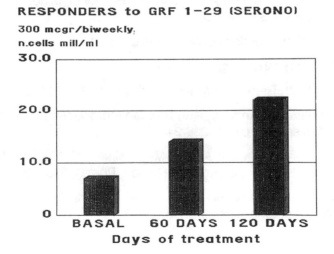

Fig. 8.
Effects of treatment with GRF (Geref Serono: 300 p. os biweekly for 4 months) on sperm concentration.

References

Barvin BN (1986). In: Andrology, Male Fertility and Sterility, JD Paulsen et al (eds), Raven Press, N.Y., 461-472.

Bellve AR and Zheng W (1989). J. Reprod. Fert., 88, 771-793.

Berry AS and Pescovits OH (1989).

Endocrinology, 123, 661-663.

Dufau ML (1988). Ann. Rew. Physiol., 50, 483-508.

Eliasson R (1983). In Male Reproduction and Fertility, A Negro-Vilar (ed), Raven Press, N.Y., 285-310.

Fabbri A, Fraioli F, Isidori A (1986). J. Endocr. Invest., 9, 521-528.

Fabbri A, Ulisse S, Bolotti M, Ridolfi M, Spera G, Dufau ML, Isidori A (1989a). In: Perspective in Andrology, M. Serio (ed), Raven Press, N.Y., 203-213.

Fabbri A, Ulisse S, Moretti C, Gnessi L, Bonifacio V, Di Luigi L, Ridolfi M and Isidori A (1989b). In: Unexplained Infertility, G Spera and L Gnessi (eds), Raven Press, N.Y., 111-120.

Fabbri A, Iannini EA, Gnessi L, Ulisse S, Moretti C, Isidori A (1989c). J. Steroid Biochem, 32, 145-150.

Fabbri A (1990). Trends in Endocr. Metab., 1, 117-120.

Isidori A (1981). Andrologia, 13, 187-198.

Isidori A (1987). Rev.Latino-Amer. Esteril. Fertil., 1, 100-110.

Isidori A (1988). In: Andrology and human reproduction, A Negro-Vilar et al (eds), Raven Press, N.Y., 236-248.

Isidori A, Alunni M, Majar A, Rufi ML, Pallotti S (1989). In: Andrologia Chirurgica in Eta' Pediatricia, Acta Medica (Roma), 218-224.

Schill WB (1986). In: Infertility: Male and Female, V Insler, B Luenfeld (eds), Churchill Livingstone, Edinburgh, 533-540.